Please remain seated until
the ride has come to a
complete stop

Please remain seated until the ride has come to a complete stop

Dave Collins Memoir

Dave Collins

Writer's Showcase

San Jose   New York   Lincoln   Shanghai

Please remain seated until the ride has come to a complete stop
Dave Collins Memoir

Writer's Showcase
an imprint of iUniverse, Inc.

For information address:
iUniverse, Inc.
5220 S. 16th St., Suite 200
Lincoln, NE 68512
www.iuniverse.com

ISBN: 0-595-21342-1

Printed in the United States of America

Courage is not something to be "mustered," but is simply there, as a natural part of those whose inner core is built on personal responsibility.

—Dave Collins

Realize the beauty of the moment, and know how lucky each of us is.

—Dave Collins

CONTENTS

Preface xi
D-Day 1
Induction 3
Sister Mary 5
Induction Continues 7
The Next Steps 11
Five Months 17
Induction–Again 20
Victims 24
Life Continues 27
Recovery 30
Results 31
Good Times 33
Induction II 34
It's Ba-a-ack 36
Induction III 38
Guinea Pig 43
Leaving on a Jet Plane 46
The Welcome 47
Welcome to Chemo 51
Into the Airlock 55
Gifts and Gratitude 57
Conditioning 59
Welcome Home 63
My Sleep Guardian 64
Life Behind the Airlock 66

Mike 70
Life Returns 73
Inching Forward 76
The Apartment 79
Life on the Outside 81
Losses 84
Gains 86
The Outside, Continued 88
Moving On 93
All Falling Around Me 95
The Long Way Home 96
The Journal 97
Epilogue 109
Afterword 111
About the Author 113

Book cover picture is a self-portrait, double-exposure, black and white photograph taken and developed by Dave Collins.

PREFACE

Everyone, it seems, has told me that I need to write a book about all of the experiences I've had as a cancer / chemotherapy / bone marrow transplant patient, and how the hell I survived the last two years. Well, here goes.

My name is Dave. I am now 33 years old. I have lived with, and beaten down, cancer (which will never, as far as I'm concerned, earn the importance of being spelled with a capital 'c'). I was first diagnosed in 1996, and have been in treatment more or less since then.

I write this foreword first as a warning: I do not, and cannot, express myself in any other way than how I perceive the world. The way I see things governs the way I write. Some of the material in this, my perception of "the ride", will undoubtedly cause some discomfort for the reader. I will not apologize for my thoughts, actions, or feelings. They are mine, they are honest, and deserve acknowledgment. I may sound a bit defensive, but this is a very personal ride. It's my life, and I am vulnerable in sharing it with you.

I should also caution you that the hideous, stunningly embarrassing lack of privacy I have repeatedly endured has resulted in the growth of thick, mortification-proof callouses. Built layer upon layer, slowly thickening over years of treatment, these callouses allow me to grab onto subjects that may cause the hands of the less-experienced to blister and peel. Do not try to grab the ropes I have climbed too tightly. Sometimes they are yanked abruptly. You have been warned.

Part of my philosophy is that one must find room for a laugh about life; without humor, the world is a very gray, uninteresting place. Without a good laugh now and then, I'd be dead. Literally. My particular brand of humor frequently delves into the forgotten humor of childhood—centering around the bathroom. If you are offended by bodily functions, revolting medical and physical procedures, filthy language, and don't appreciate a good potty joke now and then, stop here. Do not continue reading. I didn't write this to give the overly puckered, anal retentive, Mr./Ms. Manners of the world something to bitch about.

For the rest of us, climb aboard, and hang on. The ride continues.

D-DAY

I really haven't been feeling myself lately—tired, not hungry, exhausted after small exertions. Strangely, my black Labrador, Csonka, (usually stricken with separation anxiety) wants nothing to do with me. He slinks around, looks like he's afraid of me, and keeps his distance. Maybe I'll go see the doctor.

After several wasted, inconclusive visits, my condition worsens. I am eventually transferred to a hematologist / oncologist for evaluation. As I enter the crowded waiting room, I notice quite a few bald, shaky-looking cancer patients. I think to myself, "I don't belong in *here*."

Before I realize what is going on, I am face-down on an exam table with a biopsy needle stuck through the bone in my pelvis. The pain is sudden and crushing as the marrow sample is sucked out.

Impaled like a bug on a pin, I ask just what the hell they are looking for. Until now, everyone has simply said that "There may be something going on in your bone marrow." The oncologist gives me the news; I very likely have cancer—Acute Lymphoblastic Leukemia (ALL), to be exact.

"How bad is it?"

The doctor shifts uncomfortably in his chair; he has delivered this news many times, but he is clearly bothered. "Well, it's bad. But, with high-dose chemotherapy over the course of a year, we sometimes see a survival rate as high as 50%. We'll know more after the biopsy results come in."

Shit.

That's all I can think. Shit. Shit!

I drive home, dazed. I try to imagine what, *how* I am going to tell Carol, my wife. I can think of nothing that will shield her. I wish I could.

Through sobs, she tries to ask if there is a possibility of an error. I bluntly tell her that we need to accept and prepare ourselves for whatever is to come. My family seems to know that something is very wrong, because everyone calls to find out how I am feeling. I evade the question. I don't want to unnecessarily alarm anyone before the results of the biopsy. Keeping the possible diagnosis a secret is difficult; I feel like I'm lying to them. Waiting for the verdict is gut-churning. How could this *not* be a bad dream?

The doctor calls on Friday afternoon. I had told him to call as soon as the results of the biopsy arrive. He is reluctant to deliver the news over the phone, but I insist. I do, in fact, have ALL. I am to report to Mercy Hospital Monday morning to begin intense chemotherapy. Suddenly my world has become a very confusing place. I am completely spun.

Time to tell the family. In my memory, those first phone calls are the most absolutely soul-shredding things for me, the clinically damned, to do. The worst part isn't the shock and horror reflected in the voices on the other line. It's the *depth* of the shock and the *depth* of the horror that are brutal.

I realize that Csonka's avoidance of me is a sign; perhaps he can smell how close death is to me, and wisely wants to back away. He doesn't even wag his tail at me anymore. Just sits there and avoids eye contact. Not everyone that loves you can give support all the time. I have been given two days to prepare for the battle of a lifetime; a battle that may end long before the bell has sounded.

Shit.

INDUCTION

I am ready. Carol and I make our way to the hospital where we are then scuttled into a room and shown a video depicting a typical chemotherapy patient. It reminds me of the little film strips we were shown in second grade (back when stereos had turntables). Not very informative, nor very realistic. Pleasant music tinkles in the background as a guy in a lab coat babbles in a happy-go-lucky way that "You may experience some loss of appetite and nausea." Anyone who has had the pleasure of chemotherapy will appreciate the magnitude of understatement.

My blood functioning is horribly low, and I am quickly hooked up to intravenous (IV) lines and blood transfusions. My hemoglobin (the oxygen-carrying component in the blood) is so low that I should be unconscious. My platelets (the component that prevents internal or external hemorrhage by forming clots) are also dangerously low. My arms instantly turn purple as an endless succession of needles are stuck into them to take samples and to place IV lines. I am soon splayed out on the bed, with IV needles piercing veins in my left shoulder, biceps, and hand, and in my right arm and hand. Plastic bags and glass bottles of blood, platelets, as well as chemotherapy and antibiotics are pumped into me.

With IV lines attached to both sides of me, strapping me down, I can do nothing but lie on my back. My body quickly goes numb since I am unable to change positions enough to keep my circulation flowing well. The tingly, prickly feeling is frequently unbearable and excruciating. My left arm sports a swollen, bright purple, jiggly hematoma. Carol, who is quite squeamish, asks if I could *please* keep my arms under the blankets.

3

Nurses and doctors shuffle in and out, answering our questions and helping in any way they can. It is from these people that I learn the true meaning of dedication, compassion, and the good that is within us all (even lurking somewhere in the heart of the world's biggest asshole, I'm sure of it).

Four days of non-stop, high-dose chemotherapy, numerous infections due to a nonexistent immune system, and a nasty case of constipation have left me in pretty bad shape. However, in my head I know I will live. This is a speed bump. I must slow down, but I can and I will keep going.

I envision my grandmother, Meme, in my bone marrow, pissed off enough to scare the living shit out of anything in her path. She's wiping out the cancer cells with some spectacular martial arts moves that you wouldn't expect a woman of ninety to do so fluidly. The cancer cells, by the way, look kind of like the California Raisins (remember the "Heard It Through the Grapevine" commercials?), and Meme is just kicking the holy crap out of them. She's also surfing on every wave of chemo, and waving the yardstick that she once spanked me with. Those wrinkled little fucks are just *screaming* with fright, knowing they will soon be mercilessly executed by a yardstick-wielding, ninety-year-old, pissed off, surfboard-riding, Karate-kicking, great-grandmother. One by one, she lines them up for slaughter, deaf to their cries. I truly believe she was sending me her strength and resolve, and this twisted scenario is how my brain, upon receiving this energy, spit it back out to my conscious mind. I also believe that without her (as well as many, many others) I would not have made it through those first months of treatment.

Lesson: Never underestimate the power of love, prayer, God, or, for us not-so-religious people, positive energy. Allow it to surround and protect you. Take what you need and pass some on. Most importantly, know that the power and energy that flow though the universe, as well as within each of us, is always there for us to tap into when we need it.

SISTER MARY

The hospital Chaplaincy sends down a nun, whom we nickname Sister Mary (none of us can remember her real name). She is very insistent that she be given a job to do on our behalf. We are as clueless about her life experience as she is about the job we assign to her: Official Sperm Bank Research Liaison.

Her task assigned and accepted, Sister Mary goes after her goal with urgency and fervor. She makes phone calls. She researches cryogenic laboratories. She talks to insurance companies about coverage. She spends countless hours following dead-end leads. She comes in twice a day with an update on her progress. A few days later, plan in place, research done, she proudly brings in a sterile sample cup, wrapped in plastic. She hands it to me, folds her arms primly, and excitedly urges me to "produce," as she puts it.

She has no idea how a sperm sample is produced.

'Producing' a sample is about the last thing I am physically capable of doing. I have IV lines plugged into and holding down both of my arms, and I am clearly not flexible enough to try anything with my feet. I am feverish, nauseated, and incredibly weak. I cannot, no matter how insistent Sister Mary is, fathom doing *that*, in *here*, feeling like *this!* Pain, overbearing constipation, nausea, hospital food, and fever conspire to put out the fire. I tell her, "Maybe later."

She infers from this that "later" means "every couple of hours or so," and pays me a visit, cup in hand, at least three times a day for the next couple of days. She unknowingly becomes "Sister Mary Sperm Bank," and we secretly giggle after her visits. My brother, Brian a.k.a. "Pit" (whose

5

specialty is designing packaging for products) arrives with Gab (his fiancee) and my older brother Kevin. Pit proudly presents his newest creation: The Sister Mary Human Propagation Kit. Included in the cleverly designed box, printed with multitudes of upwardly-swimming sperm, are:

- 1 fluid ounce of Friction Relief Ointment (a sample pack of Astroglide)
- Visual Stimulus Media (a dirty magazine)
- Post-Sample Palm Shaving Kit (apparently my palms would grow hair despite the chemo)
- Post-Sample Eyewear (an enormously thick pair of glasses, probably from a thrift store, to combat the impending blindness)
- Patented Zip-Lock Bosom Bag (Sister Mary had apparently been advised by a local sperm bank that Carol should tuck the sample in her bra, to maintain body heat during transport).

The seal on the package reads, "Do not open in the company of the deeply religious." We all howled with laughter. So did most of the staff who weren't "deeply religious." We hid the kit under a pile of magazines when Sister Mary reliably made her thrice-daily mission to my room. We felt just a little blasphemous to be making a joke of all of this, but how could one not see the humor? She thought that all I had to do was piss into a jar, and her assignment was complete. After all, I was urinating, wasn't I? She eventually gave up, when it was clear that I couldn't (or wouldn't) comply with her simple request. We were obviously incredibly naive about how naive she was. Don't people learn about the pitfalls of self-gratification when they learn about the other stuff that will eventually result in their eternal damnation? Apparently not.

INDUCTION CONTINUES

As I am physically wasting away in the hospital bed, I keep the knowledge that Carol and I are beginning an amazing journey close at hand; I am far from being through with this life. One night, a particularly high fever has me hallucinating, and I see my bed surrounded by people, none of whom I know. They all have their hands on me, and all look very peaceful. My mother sits at the foot of the bed, cradling my feet in her hands. She is the only one who is flesh and bone, yet I realize that all these others are just as real; they are the embodiment of the wishes and hopes of those around me. I close my eyes. When I open them again, I can only see my mother. I fall asleep knowing that I am not battling this alone.

My dad, Rog, comes up to visit at least weekly. His "assignment" is to mow the lawns. He comes by after cleaning things up to say hello, but rarely stays long. Sitting in a hospital room and watching the IV lines drip is not in his realm of abilities. Doing "nothing" makes him nervous, and allows his hyperactive imagination to take him places he'd clearly rather not be. Many people are wired this way. Every individual has a different way of coping. I understand—the people who love me do everything they are capable of, and I am thankful for everything they can manage. Mowing the lawns is not just cutting grass; it is the best expression of love that my father is able to give me. I welcome it as that. He and I are both doing everything we can.

The nurses amaze me. How the hell can one see and go through what these people do on a daily basis and still have the capacity to become involved on *any* level with their patients? After two years of treatment, this simple question remains. It is amazing to me that some people have an enormous reservoir of compassion that never seems to dry up, no matter how many drought years pass. These selfless people involve themselves in others' lives, even as lives are continually snuffed out around them. Somehow, the walls that most of us would build to insulate ourselves from the pain and sorrow are never built. These heroes are rarely recognized; they simply continue to drink from their bottomless reservoirs and continue to care. Amazing.

I spend several scary days and nights hallucinating, with fevers spiking up to 104 degrees. *I* am not scared, but I manage to scare the hell out of my family. I can fuzzily remember babbling about things that I could see in a painting of a vase of flowers. Faces, women carrying babies, and someone laughing. When I was trying to show everyone (Mom, Pit, Gab, Carol) where these apparitions were, Carol and Gab's eyes got very big. All I could see was their eyes since they were wearing masks to prevent infection. In retrospect I can see what they were thinking. "Oh shit! He's completely fucked up!"

My brother, Pit, was unfazed. Noticing Carol's bug-eyed stare and rather pale complexion, he casually said, "Come on, Carolina," (his nickname for her). "Let's grab lunch." Like a zombie in a bad movie, Carol shuffled out of the room with Pit behind her.

By the time they got back, my fever-addled brain was at least somewhat back to reality. I later told Pit that he did well. He hadn't given Carol a chance to pass out or vomit. She needed to get the hell out of the room for a while, and he calmly gave her an out. One of the things that I continue to be thankful for is Pit's uncanny ability to sum up a situation, and act on the solution the instant it comes to him. He doesn't, in other words, fuck around.

One night a particularly nasty fever spikes—up to 105.1 degrees. This is the definition of "feeling like shit." I have open, swollen, festering sores blocking my nasal passages; my lips are cracked and oozing from the chemo and resulting infection; my legs have a deep, fiery ache that painkillers cannot reach. The fever has me thrashing in my sheets, completely soaked in a slick, shivery sweat. My nurse, Ed, stays in my room most of the night. I can see the concern in his wrinkling forehead and eyes, even as he reassuringly pats my head with a wet cloth. My fever continues on, unabated. Terry (another of my nurses) and Ed decide it's time for the ice. They dump buckets of ice beside me, then fold the sheet up so that I am completely encased. I am stunned not by the cold, but by the fact that I can barely feel anything. My overheated body melts the ice almost as fast as they can bring it. Convulsive shivers rack my body; uncontrollable, yet somehow comforting. I insist I will be ok, and thank them for paying so much attention to me. This does little to smooth the furrows in their brows. Finally, fever under control, and a new batch of antibiotics flooding into my veins, I sleep. Tomorrow will be a new day.

The phone rings at all hours. As word spreads, people call to express good wishes and let me know that they are thinking about me. I get calls from old high school friends, neighbors, many people I haven't spoken to in years, some I don't even know. Cards and letters arrive daily. All of the positive thoughts and energy, delivered through the phone lines or wrapped in an envelope, boost me immensely. Everyone wants to "do *something*." I tell everyone to just keep me in their thoughts; it's the best thing anyone at this point can do. I promise to keep myself open to the energy they are sending. I can *feel* their energy, lifting me from the abyss.

My blood counts begin to recover from the chemo. I am gradually weaned from transfusions and antibiotics as I begin to create my own blood once again. My nurse, Karen, arrives every morning to cheer the latest test results. Everything appears to be coming back, like the landscape after a devastating fire. Things look good. I am almost too weak to make it to the bathroom, but I steadfastly stick to my credo—I'll not be crapping in a bedpan, thank you very much.

I'm in immense pain. My legs feel as if I've torn my hamstrings and popped my Achilles tendons at the same time. The nurses, and my family, urge me to get up and walk, which I do, but don't last more than ten steps before giving in. I have, essentially, stopped eating in any significant quantity. Still, I feel incredibly blessed. Lucky. I am alive. I am loved.

Things gradually improve, but I know that I will only start to recover quickly once I am home. Real food. The doggies. My own bed with Carol beside me. The doctor agrees, and we make preparations to go home. I really don't know how I knew I would still be alive at this point, or how I knew that cancer wouldn't be what takes me out. I just knew. Maybe I'm just too stubborn to realize that I should be dead. Maybe I never looked at death as a viable option. I don't know for sure. Three weeks later, and forty pounds lighter, I am in a wheelchair, too weak to stand. Carol wheels me out and drives me home from the hospital. As we pull out of the parking lot, the weight of it all drops on me. I am winning! I have already won! I sob, raw and viscerally; too happy, too grateful to express myself in any other way. I am going *home*, and am still alive for the next stage of treatment. I am deeply indebted to the people who helped get me there.

I wonder how Csonka will react to me. I have a sense that he is able to tell if the cancer is still there better than any biopsy. I desperately need him to recognize me–to be as happy to see me as I am him. I am depending on passing the Csonka test to give myself surety.

THE NEXT STEPS

We pull into our driveway. Our neighbor, who lost her husband to cancer the previous year, is in her yard. From somewhere, I find the strength to stand, my legs on fire. I hug her, assuring her that she will *not* have to watch this happen again. Through sniffles, she tells me that she has been thinking about me. Head tilted against my shoulder, my arms around her, she pulls strength from me, even as I receive it from her, somehow creating more than had been there before. I hobble, pain invisible, back across the street, as she smiles and wipes tears from her cheeks. I cannot let her, or anyone else, down. I must live.

I still, however, haven't passed the "Csonka test."

I timidly open the door to the backyard, uneasily waiting for the verdict. Csonka comes running in, tail wagging, panting, howling at me. We are both elated! Uncle Dave is back! I have passed the test!

Much to Carol's dismay, I fall to my knees and let him jump and slobber all over me, as he pants his humidly smelly breath into my face. Carol asks if I could *please*, at *least* not let him jump on me, as I am too likely to bruise. For the moment, I am deaf. I want the drooly, clumsily bouncing celebration to continue, to enjoy every second of it. Moments like this need to be enjoyed as fully as they can. Dani, our other dog, spins happy circles around us, barking and whining for attention. It's good to be alive.

The first night back at home is strange. I am happier than I have ever been, yet I am in enormous physical pain. My esophagus is raw and literally tattered from the chemo. My legs feel as if ligaments in my thighs and calves have been mutilated with broken glass. I reject painkillers because I don't like being dizzy and the ensuing constipation is unbearable. I have not taken a decent dump in six days, and didn't feel like extending that misery any longer. I spend most of the first night in the fetal position, trying to make the pain go away. Carol spends the night awake, standing guard against the pain and the nightmares that envelop me in my fitful sleep.

It is an unbelievable shock to see myself in the mirror. There weren't any at the hospital, so I really didn't have any concept of just how far down the leukemia and subsequent chemotherapy have taken me. The first morning home, I catch a glimpse of what my body has become as I struggle to dress myself. My first flash of thought: "Who is *that?* Could that apparition staring back at me through those hollow sockets be *me?*"

I look like a corpse.

I am as skeletal and pale as a concentration-camp prisoner—my hair coming out in patches, my skin loose and sagging. My eyes and teeth look far too large for my head, and my nose is razor-thin. My legs, sickly-looking broomsticks, are attached to hugely bulbous knees. My collarbones jut out abruptly, like bony shelves above my exposed, shadowy rib-cage. My butt has disappeared, leaving only a wrinkled, empty sack where muscle once was. I am repulsed by these first images of myself, and wonder how it is that nobody around me seems to notice.

My family comes to visit during the first couple of days back at home. We take pictures to commemorate the occasion. My stomach does triple back flips when I see those pictures, even now. How the hell can one survive after looking like *that?* Makes me wonder what people were *really* thinking when they would say, "You look great!"

Bony or not, I am ecstatic to be home again. It's little things that make life so wonderful. I never thought the simple act of pissing, without alerting anyone, analyzing color, or measuring a single drop, could bring me such pleasure. I'm even marveling at the exhilarating pleasure of being able to scrape up the dog turds in the backyard. Life is good. I learn that one must sometimes lose the ability to do almost everything before they can fully appreciate and enjoy doing *anything*.

I spent the first month at home too weak even to get the mail. Normal acts took on an incredible significance. The simple act of taking a dump or eating a meal would send me back to bed for a few hours. It was a big day, activity-wise, if I crapped *and* showered without a four-hour nap in between. Still, it was one of the most fulfilling and happy thirty days of my life. To experience things coming back to me, one at a time, was very encouraging.

Recovery from grave illness is a lot like packing up everything you care about and going on a long, arduous journey. After exhausting days spent traveling, you arrive at what you think is your destination, only to discover that everything you had strapped to the roof of your car blew off at some point, far behind you. Your belongings, like your former life, are strewn along the roadway, like so many piles of forgotten trash. When you recover from the drop in your stomach, the intensely sickening feeling of loss, you climb back into the car, start the motor, and turn around, scouring the freeway for your belongings. Some things you will never see again, stolen by other motorists or buried in a ditch. Many you find and recover. Some, after looking at them with new eyes, you leave by the roadside because you realize you don't want some of that shit to be a part of your life anymore. With your new load carefully re-packed and meticulously checked, you confidently head for a different road; one that leads to a place you never knew existed.

As my strength and abilities increase, I become increasingly confident that all is well, that the chemotherapy and radiation are going to keep me alive, and that I will be alive long after the treatment has ended. I welcome each new dose—seeing it as another wave for Meme to surf, in her relentless quest to rid me of those cursed little shits—and manage to keep most of the horrendous side effects at bay. I realize that I am one of the luckiest men alive. I have an incredible wife, a close family, a wide circle of supportive and caring friends, and two drooling, happy doggies. I am free to enjoy all of them whenever I wish.

The brain radiation, weekly spinal taps, and chemo treatments suck at my strength even as I recover from the initial induction treatments, but my spirits remain high. My gains in strength are greater than the treatment can steal. Within weeks, I am able to stand long enough to do the dishes or throw the ball for the dogs. After six months, I am able to mow our small front lawn all at one time. I have regained all but ten pounds, and the chemo no longer seems to knock me down as much. I blaze through cycle after cycle, confident that everything is working. My hair starts to return three months before I am to end my chemotherapy. When I ask the doctor how, he just shrugs and says, "Sometimes that can happen."

By Thanksgiving, I am able to travel to San Jose, be with family, and attend my brother Kevin's high school football game—Kevin is the head coach, as well as a teacher. The game is the annual Thanksgiving rivalry, known as the "Big Bone" game. Whoever wins the contest gets to keep the trophy—a giant, garishly painted thighbone from some rather large animal. It is a decades-old tradition, and is attended by vast crowds of alumni and spectators. Some 7,500 people show up to cheer their team. Kevin's kids miraculously win, against a much larger, much more intimidating team. I liken my own struggle to this game; odds aren't that great, but hell, this is winnable.

Afterwards, and unbeknownst to Kevin or me, the underdog Lions all signed their winning game ball, dedicating it to me. Kevin presented me with this symbol of triumph before Thanksgiving dinner. I don't think those kids have any clue how deeply their gesture affected me. I wouldn't let them down. *Couldn't.*

Six months into treatment, I develop a frustratingly unidentifiable infection. After enduring seventy-four straight days of diarrhea and phantom fevers, and my condition on a downhill slide, I am again hospitalized. My chemotherapy is halted, giving my body a rest. I am tested and re-tested for infection, but nothing ever shows itself. Finally, I am dosed with *Vancomycin,* a new "silver bullet" antibiotic, for five days. The persistent fevers dissolve, and my energy is boosted from the many transfusions of blood, which prop up my crumbling, collapsing blood factory. The same crew of nurses that pulled me through induction happily write up my discharge papers, and I am again sent home. I still have the unexplained diarrhea, but otherwise feel well. The doctor ominously set an appointment for the next week for a colonoscopy. Yet another procedure to look forward to.

Apparently, my mischievous colon was listening in on the conversation, and decided having an unwelcome intruder unceremoniously shoved in there didn't sound like fun. The morning before my appointment, it blesses me with welcome salvation—a firm stool. The following day, I go in for my appointment. The doctor soberly asks about my symptoms. Proving that it was no fluke, my now-compliant colon graciously supplied a much-appreciated encore that very morning. I explained, "You know that awful grinding noise that mysteriously disappears when you take your car into the mechanic? Well, *my* awful grinding has disappeared, too." The doctor's serious demeanor dissolves into chuckling, and he sends me on my way. He does, however, tell me to call immediately if my symptoms reappear—"We can *always* reschedule," he assures me. My colon must have heard that as well, because it finally decided to remain well-mannered. Sometimes, the mere threat of punishment is more effective than the real thing.

Victorious, I go in for my final treatment—a four-day bout of high-dose chemotherapy, done as an inpatient. I have survived. This last dose is meaningless since there is no cancer in my system to treat. This is just a formality. I am given a dose of a drug that had been injected into my spine months earlier. When the poison reaches a certain level in my bloodstream, I will be given the antidote. It is a little disconcerting to think that I am going to need to be "rescued," which is the medical term given to the treatment, but I know I will be fine. I am determined to get through this final treatment without the problems endured during previous hospital stays. I glide through the next week, undamaged.

We are all relieved when this, the final blast, is over. I sustained no trauma, felt fine during the entire week of treatment, and am kicked out of the hospital early for good behavior. After eleven months of frequently unpleasant chemotherapy, I am freed. All the biopsies, CT scans, and blood tests confirm there is no detectable cancer in my body. Carol and I have a large party to celebrate not only the end of treatment, but the beginning of a new life.

FIVE MONTHS

For the first time in a year I am free of the ravages of chemotherapy and radiation. I quickly regain strength. Soon, I am installing landscapes, drainage systems, creating landscape designs, and doing some general construction work for a contractor. My life begins to take a new, exciting direction. It's a far cry from the tie-wearing corporate weenie I had been (although I wasn't the most enthusiastic tie-wearing corporate weenie ever to fear a layoff). I'm having fun, making a little money, and looking forward to a contractors' license and design business. Things are just taking off.

I continue to attend a weekly cancer support group. I want to be there as a symbol of hope; a physical, tangible manifestation of success. I have made fast friends within this group. Nothing bonds people quite as quickly as a shared fight for life. I want to show those new to the game that they, too, can win. Cancer is only a speed bump in their road; they may need to slow down to a crawl if it is a large one, but then punch the accelerator as soon as the rear tires are clear.

I organize and participate in rebuilding the enormous deck at our cabin. Working fourteen-hour days, we manage to finish the project in a couple of weekends, not counting my midweek deliveries of building materials. Family and friends all pitch in; the work is hard and dirty, but we are all happy to be there in the unfathomable beauty around us. I am amazed at how quickly my abilities and stamina have returned. I am the last one to drop the hammer and reach for a beer. It feels *good*.

Carol and I take a much-needed vacation, touring the U.S. and visiting our relatives throughout. I see our trip as a beginning; pouring the foundation for our new lives, the strengthening bonds to our families reinforcing the concrete. We spend three weeks laughing, eating, fishing, playing, enjoying one another's company, and creating memories together. Priceless time, well-spent with those we will always be able to depend on—family.

I send out some tentative resumes and am quickly deluged with requests for interviews, job offers, and requests for landscape design work. I am overwhelmed. Nobody even looks at the year-long gap in my work history, and apparently, nobody cares. It is hard to believe that I was ever sick. I have *never* felt better.

Then, the bruising—large, purple stains appear on my legs and back. My nose bleeds spontaneously, dripping unexpectedly down my upper lip. I ignore these symptoms for a couple of days. A couple of days spent in denial—I felt great, so there *couldn't* be a problem. I simply bruise easily now, because of the after-effects of chemo. These will fade away. I *did* scrape myself up crawling under that house. I have inhaled a lot of dust in the last week. I'll wear a dust mask to help clear up my nosebleeds. Carol and I spend an evening trying to explain the bruises to each other, nonetheless suspecting something was very wrong. A day later, I'm in my oncologist's office waiting for the lab to send up my test results. It usually takes them fifteen minutes, but today it seems to take *days*. Barbara (my chemo nurse) tells me that the Doc wants to have a few words with me. When the nurse won't deliver your test results, you suspect the news isn't good. Carol and I wait, staring mutely at the floor, too afraid of what we already know.

I've relapsed.

My white cell count has soared from a normal 4,000 to 105,000. My platelets are so low that spontaneous, fatal hemorrhage is not only possible, but common. I make an appointment for another hospital stay, for another round of high-dose induction chemotherapy.

Shit. *Shit!*

Again, I must make the dreaded phone calls, spreading grief and pain. The first is to Pit. Somehow he seems the easiest to tell first; to get my feet wet as I break the news. He promises to let Kevin, my older brother, know. The second call is to my parents. All I can think of to say is, "It's back." My mother moans as if punched in the stomach. I feel awful, because I'm the one doing the punching. The third call is to my good friend and fellow death-mocker, Louise. Louise and I met at the cancer support group I had been attending since the first round of chemotherapy. She and I had both been through the ringer, and were still kicking. We shared the same philosophy: cancer was not something to die with, but to *live* with. She was unlikely to have a meltdown over the phone, leaving me feeling helpless and at fault for the pain I was causing. Louise knew how to react, because she was *there*, walking the edge. I needed to walk that edge with someone who knew where to step.

The following morning, I go into surgery for a new central chest catheter, and chemo starts immediately. Meme dusts off her surfboard, ready to ride the next wave.

INDUCTION–AGAIN

I am now under the care of Dr. Quadro (Dr. Q, as we call him). My previous oncologist has changed practices. We are disturbed to learn that many things, such as a marrow typing for myself and family, should have been done while I was in remission. We hadn't been informed of this precaution. A search of the National Bone Marrow Registry could (should) have been completed already, but was, apparently, overlooked because of HMO cost-cutting. They saved $147 by not testing me. The way I see it, those fucking bastards pushed me in front of a bus because I was standing on some money, and they wanted it.

I am pissed.

Never again will I allow some pencil-pushing insurance shithead dictate the terms of MY treatment. It's my *life*, and I wasn't going to let a couple of measly (hundred thousand) dollars get in my way. How the *fuck* can these "people" be so inhuman as to place a monetary value on my *life*? They don't even know me. I make it a point from this day forward, to ask every question, including questions like, "Is this decision determined by money, or by my best interests?" I learn to ask, regardless of how my questions may be interpreted. At this point, I am in no mood to worry about some cost-cutting MBA asshole getting offended. I ask. I offend. Tough shit.

Fortunately, I am now in the hands of a very aggressive doctor who, for lack of a better term, doesn't give a rat's ass about getting a bonus from the HMO for keeping his level of care low. He cares about people, not dollars. He goes after everything with an enthusiasm that surprises me. He is optimistic, yet realistic. I feel sure that any decisions we make together (Carol, me, and Dr. Q) will be in my best interests.

Occasionally, during remission, I wondered if I would have the same interest in life, the same fight left in me, if I were to relapse. I didn't know if I could find another well that still held water. Faced with what I am now, I realize that if I dig deeply and tirelessly, more water can be found—cold, pure, and revitalizing. I am surprised to find hidden new reserves, below the thick bedrock, cold and brimming, from which I can drink and grow strong. I arrive at the hospital fully prepared. I will not lose the weight. I will not lose the strength. I will go into remission, go to San Francisco, and receive an autologous Bone Marrow Transplant. I will live.

VePesid. Mitoxantrone. Daunorubicin. The latest toxic brew to make its way through my veins. Mitoxantrone turns my piss the color of window cleaner. Bright blue. Nurses administer these chemicals wearing rubber gloves, gowns, and goggles. After the chemo is pumped into me, all of their protective gear goes into a special hazardous waste container. I wonder what is so dangerous about what is now coursing through my system, but nevertheless ask the nurses to completely drain each infusion. I want every last drop. I down an average of four gallons of water every 24 hours. I don't want the chemo to settle in my liver or kidneys and cause failure. I have enough problems.

I am, blessedly, feeling good through the chemo. We have been keeping the food intake high by avoiding anything that is brewed in the hospital's kitchen. The nurses soon realize that if they bother to bring in my tray, it will be swiftly, consistently rejected. Occasionally, I do take a morbidly curious peek at what I would be trying to choke down if it weren't for the blessing of Carol and her thrice daily food runs: Bright orange chicken thingies, miserably bathing in their own congealed juices; mushy vegetables, once colorful but cooked to a uniform gray; soggy dinner rolls sweating in their chemical-smelling cellophane wrappers stare back at me when the nurses smirkingly lift the lids on these gastronomical nightmares. I unlock one secret to survival during chemo—don't eat hospital food. It may be what really makes patients sick.

I regularly walk around the hospital wing, IV pole in tow; I have developed great skill in maneuvering it through the crowded halls. I witness grim realities during these walks. Each room I pass has a different story. Life and death hover at every doorway, each waiting to be beckoned in. Occasionally (usually very late at night), there is a body, encased in a black zippered bag, waiting anonymously in the hallway. Who loved these people? Who did these people love? What are they waiting for? Having left their bodies, do they look back at the black, androgynous lump on the gurney and see themselves? Did they choose death, or did death choose them? Is somebody, somewhere, mourning their passing, or did they die lonely and unnoticed, the ripples of their existence diminishing, unseen? I walk and I wonder. I visualize death, calling me forward, scythe at the ready; when I am close enough to smell his rotten, curdled breath, I boot that bony bastard in the nuts.

The woman in the room next to me appears to be on her way out. She is maybe 35, and her cancer is out of control. Three puffy-eyed generations gather to hold vigil outside her door. Often, when I can't sleep, I must dodge the waiting masses, sleeping underfoot like exhausted dogs. As I maneuver the IV around them, I try not to imagine my family out there, sadly holding the candle, as my flame is snuffed out.

I know the minute that she dies. Unbelieving moans of grief and deep, wrenching sobs echo through the thick, cold walls. Julie, my nurse, comes in to check vitals, closing the door on the scene behind her. She is visibly, acutely affected, tears bubbling in her eyes, yet she resolutely goes on with the business at hand, checking my vital signs. I stop her, and invite her to sit down and let it all settle for a while. She sits heavily, driven down by the weight of emotion; her arms hang limply at her sides, eyes wide and staring. Finally, she manages a deep, shaking breath, looks me in the eye, and thanks me, telling me she appreciates my understanding, as well as the chance to decompress. Allie comes in. He, too, is seeking refuge; a place where he knows his feelings don't need to be squelched. He chokingly tells us, "She told me ten minutes ago. She said, 'I'm going to die now.' Before I could get back with her meds, she was gone." Unaware, he still holds the unused cup of pills, as if still wanting *someone* to give them to. I am touched that they have become this close to me, to share their anguish with me, to make room in their hearts to include me. I suspect I am just one of many, and the woman next door was too.

VICTIMS

The hospital's chaplaincy seems confused as to what to do with me. Representatives stop by daily to ask if I have made my peace with God, if I have been forgiven. They paradoxically seem obsessed with death, not with life. It's almost as if they are trying to dampen my spirits, coming into my room with weepy-eyed, "I really feel sorry for you" expressions on their faces. They say things like, "You must really be depressed to be in this horrible condition" and call my life a "tragedy." They ask who I blame. One woman asks how I will feel, what I would turn to, if all treatments fail, "as they often do." Good grief, this is supposed to be *uplifting?* I would have to be in a dark, bottomless, free-fall for this kind of bullshit to do me any good. I can only guess that this must work for some people, but it certainly doesn't work for me.

They essentially beg me to assume the victim role, which I'll have nothing to do with. I have *never* questioned the enormous blessings, freely given to me, in my life. What the hell gives me the right to question the bad? I am prodded to complain, to whine, to gripe, to boo-hoo about my "tragic plight." I tell them with a smile, "I'm still here, still alive, and there are a hell of a lot of people out there worse off than I am." They appear baffled; they shake their heads as they leave my room, maybe convincing themselves I have not accepted the possibility of my own death. I *know* I have, but I'm not checking-out bitching about how unfair everything is, how I got the shaft, how I drew the short straw.

A victim's initial response is blame, followed closely by enduring self-pity. Refusal to take something from the experience and move on shows that a victim simply refuses responsibility. I am not, by any means, saying that people are responsible for or deserve some of the terrible things that happen to them. If you have been raped, for example, you are *obviously* not responsible for the heinous act. What you *are* responsible for is *what happens next.*

Too many people use jarring life experiences as a crutch; an excuse for their drug problem, financial woes, you name it. They can see good if it is the *only* thing there. Personal responsibility, and the strength it requires to maintain, provide the foundation to support the creation of something wondrous. It gives each of us, if willing, the ability to shake life's traumas and create something wonderful from *everything*, not just the good stuff. To truly experience life one must draw from the pool of it all including, and especially, the ugly or difficult. The biggest cop-out in the world is only to see beauty in something beautiful. Life is about extracting what is meaningful from the ugly and unpleasant.

There are a few things in my life now that are sure: I never asked for this disease; I don't deserve to have this disease; I want to put this disease far back in my rearview mirror. I bristle at the thought of anyone looking at me with pity, and it makes me sick to think that anyone would ever call me a victim of anything (especially cancer). I have so much good in my life; cancer has only served to accentuate and highlight that fact. Send me all of the good energy that you can, but save pity for someone who wants it.

Life has been unusually good to me. Just because I plan to stick around and enjoy the ride for a little while doesn't mean I can't fathom death as a part of life. Life *causes* death, which causes life all over again. Nothing really ends. *"Every new beginning comes from some other beginning's end."* (Semisonic, from *Closing Time)*

I am not involved with organized religion, and do not accept the concept that you can go through life as a complete asshole, beg forgiveness, be forgiven, and magically be transformed into a good person simply because you fear going to hell. The motivation for being a genuinely good person, in my beliefs, is to *be* a genuinely good person. I do not subscribe to the 'extra reward if you do good things' theory; that is how people train their pets not to shit on the carpet. Being honest, tolerant, loving, giving, and loyal carries its own rewards, to be enjoyed and shared during *this* life, and carried on to the next.

LIFE CONTINUES

Sleeping during a hospital stay is an unrealistic goal. To combat the sometimes brutal and depressing sounds that creep under my door and steal my sleep, I develop a unique system. Late at night, when the sounds of patients screaming in pain or fright, having infections suctioned, and moaning in delirium seem to be at their peak, I strap on the headphones. Not pleasant, comforting music, but fast, loud, blasphemous, and angry. I am here to kick the shit out of something. This is *no* place for sappy crooning or calming instrumentals. It is, however, a perfect venue for the enraged, disaffected rantings of the seriously disturbed. Volume up as high as it will go, I find my peace in the violence and hostility reflected in the music and lyrics. At times I wake up with headphones still on, still at high volume, only it's hours later. A few times, I accidentally pull the headphone jack out as I sleep, which brings the night nurses running. Nothing compares to the mayhem created by some unknown, pissed-off, marginally pubescent punk-rock band screaming maximum-volume obscenities at three A.M. I certainly did my share to add to the nighttime ambiance.

When my immune system finally reaches rock bottom, I am sequestered to my room, to avoid the dangerously germ-laden hallways. I use a portable stairstepper to keep the blood flowing, and exhaust my body enough to sleep when my overactive brain won't let me rest. I paste pictures and cards all over the room, to be reminded of what life once was, and can be again. Louise brings her beautiful, gregarious granddaughter, eight-year-old Stephanie, to visit. Stephanie is a veteran hospital visitor, and has with her a drawing that she made specifically for me. It is a flower, vividly colorful and grinning. I tape it up where I can see it easily. It epitomizes optimism and happiness. I still have it.

Visitors from the cancer group come by daily: Carson always brings a gift, even as I insist that she doesn't need to; Lem, who is like Yoda—he opens his mouth and something wise and thoughtful comes out; Diana brings a 'State Fair' T-shirt along with her smile; and Charlotte, quite possibly the toughest of the group—fourteen *years* of fighting metastatic bone cancer, with her husband Hubert at her side. I am supported. I am thriving. I will live.

Many of the nurses stop in to see us, even if they aren't assigned to me. Karen, one of my most fervent supporters, comes in every day to check my progress. She has become a part of my life, as have many others. I feel a kinship with all of them. They have, over the months of treatment, become family; my own private cheerleading squad. I remain in awe of their acceptance of tragedy, and of their capacity to continually reach out, even as their hands and hearts are being cut and injured.

Coincidentally, a lymphoma patient, Chris, is in the same wing, also in relapse. We had undergone the same treatment with the same doctor, and both were readmitted in relapse within the same week. All I knew about him was that he was twenty years old, as hairless as I was, and looking at a bone marrow transplant. We'd crossed paths a few times, and nodded at each other as we went to chemotherapy every week. I went down the hall, IV in tow, and introduced myself formally. As it turned out, we both needed some company.

I soon became kind of a coach, trying to help him through his induction. He was having it pretty rough. Thankfully, I wasn't. I would get him out of bed to walk, bring him food from the refrigerator (At this point, none of the nurses bothered to scoot me or Carol out of the "employees only" area.) He made some progress, but battled some serious side effects. I got to know his mother. His father, back from a business trip, knocked on my door one night, and with tears in his eyes, thanked me for all I was doing. I was doing what also helped me, so I told him I felt his thanks were unnecessary.

One day, when I went to see how Chris was doing, he unblinkingly told me that he had found a new tumor. The lymphoma had returned. He was ineligible for a transplant. He was going home to spend his remaining days with family around him. He seemed relieved; the dense, crushing weight of the fight lifted, he was at peace.

I shook his hand, looked into his eyes, and couldn't find anything to say. I just looked, and he looked back. His strength and peace became mine. I gave his mother a long, rocking hug as she squinted tears onto my shoulder. They wished Carol and me the best. I looked back as we left his room: the photograph my mind took is one reflecting both peace and grief. Chris was smiling slightly and nodding, looking tired. Finished. At peace. He knew he did the absolute best he could, and would live (and die) with that knowledge. And his mother, already sitting down, swollen eyes staring at the floor; knowing she is losing her son and cannot intervene. Not, perhaps, believing she will be able to go on. I turned from this scene and walked out.

I never saw them again.

RECOVERY

My body very quickly recovers from the chemo, which Dr. Q finds amazing. I have no infections, no fevers, no weight loss, and am soon walking around the neighborhood, instead of the hallways or the stairstepper. We are all confident that this re-induction worked, and I would be off to San Francisco to get an autologous bone marrow transplant.

After twenty-eight days in the hospital, I am released to go home and continue recovery. Within a week, I undergo another biopsy. I tell everyone that the pain from these isn't bad, because it's short-lived. Ohholymotherfuckinghell it's painful, for a *long* ten minutes. I grit my teeth, not moving, not daring to flinch as the sharp jolts of pain explode in my hip, spreading with electric speed down my legs. There is a large (knitting needle) aspirating syringe sucking marrow out of my pelvis. I can't imagine the pain if I were to suddenly move while the doc has a hold of that thing. Drilling into the bone isn't the rough part; it's the horrible, imploding feeling that bears down when the sample is sucked out. Results of the painfully surrendered bone marrow will be available in the next couple of days. He'll call us the minute the lab gets back to him. We wait. Nothing more can be done. What comes will come.

RESULTS

I get the call. I know the second he says, "Hello, Dave. I've got your results." I can *feel* his unease through the phone line. "They aren't really good. It may be that we took the biopsy too early, but I really don't think so."

So that's it. The cancer hasn't even paused for breath. We call San Francisco to discuss with the doctors what to do next. Carol and I travel to UCSF, confused and lost in its crowded hallways. It is the first time that we actually see the facility, so far from home, in which I am to undergo my transplant. We have been forewarned that the doctor at UCSF has a blunt, rather cynical bedside manner. I assure Dr. Q that there isn't much he can tell us that we don't already know. In the business of cancer treatment, it would be almost impossible to remain optimistic with death so close all the time.

Upon meeting the doctor, I do not find him to be pessimistic or cynical—it is much worse than that. He is condescending and domineering. He says, in a tone one might use to explain to a small child, "You are still in relapse. This is bad. *Very* bad."

My head says, "No shit! You think I don't know that?" but my mouth says, "I know. I need to know what options I have to induce remission." He begins a long, detailed lecture about percentages and possibilities for treatments that do not apply to me. Carol interrupts him, saying, "We already know Dave's brothers aren't a match. We need to know what *else* could be done."

He turns quickly and glares at her. His look, one of scorn and undisguised superiority, stands my hair on end. He continues his one-sided

31

lecture, as if Carol has never spoken, still looking at her with eyes that say, "*I'm* the expert. *You* keep your mouth shut when I speak. *Your* opinion is not valid." My hackles are up. I feel the need to protect Carol, to smack this self-important asshole in the face, to let him know that by ignoring us, he is ruining my ability to trust him with anything, especially my life. I cannot trust anyone that refuses to consider me as an individual. I wonder how many other patients, each with differing diseases and treatment options, have endured this lecture; no doubt repeated hundreds of times, practiced and perfected, and *never* to be interrupted. I wait patiently for him to finish his little diatribe, somewhere knowing that I never want to rely on him for anything. He has earned his place on my shit list, right below the leukemia itself. He has affected my chances, simply by treating me and Carol as if we don't matter.

It is decided that I undergo a different induction therapy, this one very aggressive. I would need at least three weeks to recover between the last dose and the next to help avoid major organ trauma. Plan in place, we make our way through the next weeks.

GOOD TIMES

As luck would have it, Pit and Gab's wedding, and the Bachelor party, are planned right in the middle of this break, and I am able to attend both. I am, after all, the best man. The bachelor party is a big, cigar-smoking, poker-playing, fishing-rod-casting, greasy rib-eating beer-fest up in the mountains, at our cabin. I am pale, bald, and shivery, but manage to have a great time. People treat me not as if I'm doomed, but like I'm just another guy at a party. I get to forget, for the moment, that I have cancer. God, it's refreshing.

I fish. I play poker. I laugh. A lot. I pee from high places. I lose plenty of dignity at the horseshoe pit. I have a beer or two. I am allowed to, once again, feel normal; I'm no different than anyone else there, and nobody makes it a point to tell me differently. I'll say it again—God, it's refreshing.

Months before, I had secretly thought to myself, "I've got to live long enough to attend the wedding. I owe it to the people who have helped get me this far. I *will* live until then and beyond. I must."

INDUCTION II

It's now late September. Another four days' worth of chemotherapy is pumped into my veins. This time, it is ara-C, a drug that I have had before, but never in a dose this high. My confidence in my ability to manage the side effects is high. I have been here before, and have impressed the local medical community with my ability to withstand the rigors of high dose chemotherapy. I will buzz through this round, with the goal of remission, get the auto BMT, and come back home a month or so later. Life will be different, but I am excited about getting it started again. The nurses at Mercy slip a few times, saying it's great to have me back, then fall into avalanches of apologies. I know what they mean, and leave it at that. The hospital has become a second home, they have become part of my family. It's always nice to be welcomed home.

My mother (M.A.) calls me at the hospital. She's on her way to the airport; Meme has been in a car accident, and has not regained consciousness. Her chances are not good. M.A. is flying to Indiana, possibly (likely) to say goodbye. I can feel Meme's strength, urging me forward, sending me power over my struggle, even as she is now in one of her own.

Days later, kept alive on a respirator (against her wishes), she unexpectedly regains consciousness. Doctors have determined, in the meantime, that she is paralyzed from the neck down and would have to remain on the respirator for the rest of her life. She mouths, "I don't see what all the fuss is about. I probably wouldn't have lived much longer anyway. It's really OK to let me go now."

I can only sit passively on the sidelines, in my own hospital room, numb and emotionless. I had reached my capacity for life-and-death struggles, and could not be involved. I was inert, dormant; unable to put anything into motion, and unable to slow anything that was already moving. I was too tired, too burdened to help her as she had helped me. My inability to *do*, to *feel* anything still stabs me with sharp barbs of guilt.

Meme's faith, energy, and strength had helped keep me alive; her role in my twisted visualization during chemotherapy was one of the elements that let the chemo work. Meme died peacefully, surrounded by people who loved her. I hope she knew that if I had the power, I would have been there, too. Somehow, her death was comforting; she would welcome me if I ran out of options.

Within the same week, my brother's second child, Anjelica, is born, healthy and happy. The cyclic nature of life, energy, and the universe does not escape me. I know we all must die at some point, to be reborn to a different existence. I am further comforted by this new miracle, entering our lives, and helping us to celebrate not only her fresh, new life, so full of possibilities, but Meme's spent life, brimming with the possibilities that were so blessedly and generously fulfilled.

It's Ba-a-ack

I am again released from the hospital, after a little more than a month of recovery from the induction. I am glad to be out, but I know there is much ahead of me, so I don't put energy into celebrating. I have a feeling I may need a little extra very soon. Carol, too, is subdued as we pack up the stairstepper, and other equipment she has become so used to carting back and forth. We wait for another week at home for my blood counts to recover completely.

My recovering blood counts begin to look a little funky. I am concerned with my white blood cell count. It's a little too high for my liking, and climbing rapidly. In two days, it has tripled, and I don't feel like this is a good sign. I spend my energy having as much fun as I can, as I suspect that my time may be short.

Rog, Kevin (Skip) and Pit all drive up to meet me at a fishing hole on the Delta, and we spend a fun day out fishing (but not necessarily catching). I am reluctant to discuss any of the recent test results, as I would rather have a day of relative fun versus a day of nervous speculation. There is always (too much) time wasted on speculation, which always invents a more frightening story than reality. Even when the news is the worst it can be, reality is easier to deal with than the impenetrable unknown. I keep my answers vague, telling them that it's still too early to make any judgments; we'd probably know next week, maybe later. I feel like a liar, but I am not interested in wasting my time mourning anything. Why ruin a good time? I'm not dead yet.

Looking at the numbers, and the geometric increases of the past two days, Carol, Dr. Q, and I know that the higher dose didn't work. We have an appointment at UCSF, to discuss transplant options. Carol and I presume I have run out of possibilities and imagine we will be told to give up. Strangely, the night before the appointment, and its concurrent death sentence, is not spent in mourning. Carol and I meander the streets surrounding the hospital, eat a wonderful dinner, and spend the evening in an ethereal, foggy euphoria. Enjoying the hour, the minute, the *second*. We fully expected a wave goodbye to greet us in the morning, yet we were unafraid.

The doctor at UCSF surprises us, happily. Although he doesn't hold much hope, he tells us that he's willing to authorize a dose of chemo that is so high that I "may not live through the side effects," but has a *chance* of killing off my multi-agent resistant leukemia. He calls Dr. Q, is unable to reach him, and gives us the information to relay instead. We are to go straight to the hospital in Sacramento for immediate treatment.

We stop, halfway home, and call Dr. Q from a gas station. It's after 5:00, but he'll meet us at the hospital. I read to him the details of the treatment. His dismay at the high dose is apparent, but he realizes this will be my last and only hope. I have a feeling that this will be the one. It will work. I will live.

INDUCTION III

We arrive at the hospital, ready for battle. The next day, Carol brings in the stairstepper, menus from local restaurants, CD player for late-night angry punk played at high volume, and the thoughts and prayers of the people in our lives with us. I'm not dead yet. I am willfully, *violently* alive.

I am infused with the first half of the chemotherapy, but the pharmacist puts a hold on the rest of it; he believes the dosage to be a mistake. It must be, because it's three times the dose ever administered by this hospital. Dr. Q, unfortunately, left town that evening, and cannot be reached. Repeated pages to UCSF go unanswered. I spend the entire night wide awake, demanding that I get the full dose, bitching to anyone who opened my door, and generally making a pain in the ass of myself. I repeatedly demand to speak to the pharmacist, to give him the ass-chewing that he deserves for getting in the way. I am livid—my last chance at life is being flushed down the shitter by an idiot pharmacist who has no fucking clue about me. I want to grab him by the neck and shake him until he hands me the rest of the dose. It's *mine*, goddammit.

My incessant bitching finally pays off, and I am given the second half of the dosage. I later recognize that the pharmacy was acting in what would normally be my best interests. Doctors make mistakes in dosages all the time. Part of their job is to catch potential screw-ups and help correct them. "He must have meant three grams, not *eight*…hell, that's potentially a lethal dose."

Lethal or not, the chemo is pumped into me. My upwardly-mobile leukemia is rudely slapped down, hopefully for good. The rest of my body, however, takes a good portion of the chemotherapy's punch. The ride once again gets bumpy. Diarrhea is oppressively constant. Sometimes, I just stay on the toilet because I know there will be another blast coming along in five minutes or so. My appetite evaporates, but I force down foul-tasting food nonetheless. Ravaging, unsympathetic fevers strike, and after four hours of ruthlessly ascending temperature, I am once again packed in ice. Carol brings in rubber gloves, stuffed with ice, and applies them to my neck, armpits, and groin. Apparently, the sight of me lying on the bed, with two white, swollen 'hands' encircling my crotch, is too much for Carol and the nurses. They share a tension-breaking laugh at my expense. I don't mind too much. If I had felt a little better, chances are good that I'd join them, if not add a few juvenile touches of my own. My fever is completely unaffected, and soon I am covered in ice-filled plastic bags, pilfered from the janitorial-supplies room. Still, no effect. The nurses hesitatingly call the ICU, asking about available bed space. I feel the jagged leading edge of fear, and I worry about Carol. I wonder if she can sit by and watch this. For the first time, I feel myself being sucked downward; spiraling in a free-fall. All I can do is all I can do, and I'm close to that limit.

Carol is all business. She has a determined, emotionless look on her face; the face of a teacher about to punish a disruptive student. She is *not* going to fuck around with this. She calmly brings in buckets of ice, wraps the ice in plastic, and continues to bury me in its unreachable coldness. My temperature climbs upward, unabated. Soon, worried-looking nurses (Aime, Allie, and Abe) bring a refrigerated pad from another floor, and set it at fifty degrees. I lie on top of it, and Carol replaces my frigid cocoon. I redefine my own concept of "feeling like shit." My fever, edging toward 105 degrees, finally begins to respond. I shake convulsively, but feel almost human as it drops below 102. I eat some yogurt, the first food for the day. The resulting energy I gain is almost instantaneous. Aime stops in, syringe in hand, "Anyone care for some Ativan and maybe a little nap?"

I eagerly nod affirmative—relieved, exhausted. With the help of the Ativan, I am sure to sleep tonight. Carol, job completed, drives home to get her own dose of much-deserved rest. My admiration of her and her strength grows every day. It's now 2 AM, twelve hours after the initial fever struck. I wonder if Carol can rest tonight. Somehow, I know she won't. She was on autopilot for twelve hours, and she would have to decompress. She knows as well as I do how close I was. God, I'm tired. As the Ativan pulls its hazy curtain over me, I drift into sleep.

I am awakened in the early morning by Velma, often my nighttime nurse. We know each other pretty well by now, as I have spent about four months of my life under her nightly watch. She carefully sits at my bedside, drawing vial after vial of blood for the daily battery of tests. As she fondly brushes my shiny, hairless scalp, she sternly orders me not to spike another fever, waggling her finger like a mother scolding a mischievous child. Thankfully, I am able to comply.

Within the first week, my white blood cell count quickly drops to zero, and stays there. My other blood counts are maintained through transfusions. If my white cells don't start to rebound, I am going to die. The marrow would be completely destroyed beyond any treatment. After another 2 weeks, my marrow finally shows signs of life. I (as well as everyone else) breathe a sigh of relief. Hopefully, my leukemia is gone and I can get on with the transplant.

During my present stay, Dr. Q goes on vacation. Another oncologist fills in for him. He stops by while doing rounds, asks me how I feel, and leaves. Two hours later, my nurse (Tina) comes in, asking me if I *really* need the feeding tube and nutritional supplements. Apparently, the doctor, upon listening to me say that I was fine and that everything was going well, ordered all kinds of strange and seemingly incongruous infusions, painkillers, and treatments. He had not consulted or discussed anything with me. I ask to see the chart, and read the orders. Sure enough, there is an entire list of treatments ordered that I could see no good reason for me to undertake. I refuse all of them, and plan to have a few words with him in the morning. I *will* be involved in any decision made about my care, and will *not* be randomly, carelessly treated by an uninvolved doctor. You, Mr. Doctor, are not a veterinarian, so don't treat me like I'm a fucking dog, unaware and unable to make decisions about my own care.

Around lunch, he knocks on my door, and asks why I refused treatment. I inform him that he needs to discuss any future orders regarding my care with me. I am ultimately responsible for my life, and I view his role as the expert adviser, not the decision maker. It is clear that he is surprised by this, but he makes little comment. I tell him that I hope he learned something to use in the future; patients are individuals that may want a say in what gets plugged into them. He apologizes, and makes a hasty retreat. Tina sneaks in minutes later, wanting details and applauding as I tell her what I told him.

About the time my immune system is at its lowest, I develop a new symptom, one that will greatly increase my embarrassment-tolerance level. I am stricken with a nasty case of 'roids. Nine times a day, sometimes more, my anus is the hotly debated topic of discussion, guests or not. After all the hospital time I've done, the line that defines what is embarrassing for most people to talk about in any setting has become somewhat blurred for me. Questions like, "What does your bottom look like?", "Is your bottom swollen?", "Does your bottom hurt when you make a BM?" are relentlessly thrown at me. I field the barrage of questions with one simple answer: "My asshole hurts." I refuse to use the word "bottom" to refer to my bunghole. I'm not in kindergarten anymore (at least not physically).

When it was clear that the problem "down there" was not going away, and was going to need treatment of some kind, it became obvious that none of the team was highly motivated to get in there and take a peek. My anus was one hell of a hot potato, and I pictured my concerned health-care team furtively playing 'rock, scissors, paper' outside my door, to determine who would receive the dubious honor of strappin' on the gloves and spreadin' my swollen, painful cheeks. One nurse urged Carol to look, then make a full report later. I guess she chose 'rock' to someone else's 'paper', and was hoping for an easy way out. Another nurse, apologetically explaining her lack of zeal, told me it was more embarrassing for *them* with younger patients. Many of the older ones were delirious, and didn't know the difference. Every day, I wondered who would be the unfortunate soul, tragically singled out as the loser of the game. Dr. Q was clearly winning most of these contests, because he kept saying, "Someone will check on it later."

Soon, all of the nurses (and my infectious disease specialist) who had been afflicted with the dreaded rectal malaise during their pregnancies were having a powwow in my room, openly discussing what worked best for them. Four women surrounding me, enthusiastically sharing a stirring conversation about what magic potion cured each of their angry anuses, and what may help mine. Very nice. Various treatments were hotly debated. Sits baths. Prep-H. Teething cream (ostensibly to numb the pain). Dr. Barger, the infectious disease specialist, had the best advice of all, if not the most entertaining. She maintains a very prim, all-business exterior, so I was understandably shocked when she urged me to soak a sponge in iced Witch Hazel, and (direct quote) "cram it in my butt-crack." She completed her advice with an exaggerated physical depiction of said act. The other nurses nodded eagerly in agreement, and soon *I* was crammin' Witch Hazel in my butt-crack.

The embarrassment line marches onward and outward, barely visible on the faraway horizon. You have, ad nauseam, been warned.

A couple of weeks later, rectum blissfully on the mend, I am again released from the hospital. My bone marrow needs a little more time to recover before accurate testing can be done, so we pack up and head home. When we arrive, I give the doggies plenty of extra attention, as I have missed them as much as they missed me.

Forty-two days have gone by since the frantic phone call to Dr. Q from the noisy gas station along Interstate 80. I undergo another bone marrow biopsy, and impatiently wait for the results to come in. They finally arrive. I am not in remission. I have run out of options. I call UCSF, and my doctor there tells me, "It's a statistical zero that you will be treatable. You probably have a few weeks. We've done all we can."

Shit. *Shit!*

GUINEA PIG

There is no such thing as try; there is do and there is do not.
　　　　—Yoda, a long time ago in a galaxy far, far away.

Despite everything, I feel physically and mentally fine. I can take a few more on the chin before I go down. I'd much rather take the shots standing up. Getting kicked in the ribs while you're lying down is no way to go out. This shit better KO me, or I'm going to keep coming at it. I realize that there is a time and place to quit, to give up. I accept that. But I am not there yet. At the very least, I want to continue fighting in the hopes that something useful can be learned to pass on to the next patient.

Dr. Q is right behind me. He says, "I don't think your chances are good, but you are in amazingly good shape. *I* think you should keep going. Let's find you an experimental treatment or clinical trial. You would be a perfect study subject." I like this about him. He can spot a few stars, even on the cloudiest nights. He has contacted a few major cancer centers looking for an experimental treatment to enroll me in. We ask if we can be of help during this search, and he's all for it. The fun begins.

We follow lead after lead, oblivious to hours, time zones, or our own need for sleep. We ferret a few viable options; among the most promising are umbilical cord blood cell transplants, and monoclonal antibodies. Carol and I have researched the various forms of and treatments for leukemia exhaustively; I am often asked where I practice oncology, or who my patient is, and am greeted with stunned silence when I tell them that *I* am the patient. Carol has the same experience. I often hear her patiently explaining, "No, I'm his wife. No, I'm not a doctor. No, his doctor didn't tell me to call you. We are conducting our own search. He has recurrent, refractory, pre-B cell acute lymphoblastic leukemia. No, he does not exhibit the Philadelphia chromosome. No, he has no genetically-linked abnormalities. Yes, his peripheral blast count is above 100,000. He has undergone the Linker protocol, VP-16/ mitoxantrone induction, ara-C induction, and 8 grams of cyclophosphamide. No, he has not reached his lifetime limit for adriamycin. No, he is home with me, and he feels fine."

We know what we are doing. One can process *massive* amounts of information when motivated to learn. It is a good thing that they treat us like doctors. We have no time to play any games. The bullshit, condescension, concern for the patient's feelings, and false hope are eliminated when two physicians speak. We need baggage-free information, and that is what we are receiving. What we are *demanding*.

We are, at this point, rejecting any experiments that rely solely on chemotherapy. I had driven that road past the pavement, into the dirt, to where it ends in the thickly-growing trees. We need to find new roads, many of which may be just around the next corner. We sign up for a registry search, to look for a possible match on the umbilical cord transplant list. A few centers on the East Coast had experimented with this type of transplant with adults, but found most success with children. Adults, they guessed, may need larger quantities of cells to transplant than an umbilical cord could supply. However, I may be a good candidate, as my body mass is only a little greater than the largest successful pediatric case. I am given a five-percent chance with this option. It sure beats zero. Twenty-six adults have undergone this treatment. If the 5% rule has been culled from their success, there is still at least one of them out there, still alive. I could very easily make it two. Given the time, I would like to talk to the lone survivor, to compare notes. As the cord-blood coordinators scour the registry for an umbilical cord match, we continue our own search, knowing that there is more to explore, and that time is an expensive luxury, not to be wasted.

The hours buzz by.

On day five of frantic, all-hours searching the Internet, the NCI clinical trials listing, and the Leukemia Society, Carol and I hit pay dirt.

Carol and I are extremely grateful that some hope remains. We have managed to transform a "statistical zero" into a fighter once again. I couldn't wait to get back in the ring. I am the 100-to-1 shot, but I like the odds—probably because I have chosen to ignore them. They don't necessarily apply to me.

In the interest of haste, I went to Dr. Q's office to photocopy my chart and get my most recent slides and X-rays. Dr. Q, although busy with patients, stopped me in the halls to wish me the best. I could see in his eyes that he believed he was looking at a dead man. I have seen that look in many eyes. Nurses, several doctors, friends, neighbors. One place that I haven't seen those eyes is in the mirror.

I tell Dr. Q that I know what I'm up against, but am very excited to be given another chance. Maybe something they can learn from me will save the next guy. I couldn't lose. I thank him for all he had done, and say, "If it weren't for your help, I'd be screwed." His chin quivers a little, then he surprises me with his unabashed, uncensored honesty. "I think you might be screwed anyway, Dave, but I will pray for you." I am touched that he respects me enough to be so candid.

I again tell him, "We both know that this is likely not to work. Worst case, what is learned from me will help someone else."

His eyes begin to swim; he reaches for and hugs me. Saying goodbye. I hug him back; we both wonder if it won't be the last time.

Walking out of the clinic, Barbara and the other staff give me tearful hugs and good wishes—ammunition to be used in future battles. I pass the receptionist, who is crying and waving goodbye. It is hard for me to believe how entwined all of these wonderful people have become in my life. They will *all* learn from me. I will live.

LEAVING ON A JET PLANE

I just want to fly, put your arms around me baby,
put your arms around me baby.

—Sugar Ray, from song "Fly."

We made contact with the bone marrow clinic in South Carolina on Friday. By Saturday, we decided that this treatment was the one. Tuesday, we boarded the plane. Insurance had yet to approve my treatment. We drove to San Jose, where my family lives, to drop the doggies off, pick up Pit and M.A., and go to the airport early the next morning. My dad (Rog) says goodbye. There is desperation in his voice, his eyes, and his hug. It may be the last one he will give to or receive from his middle son. I try to reassure him, saying, "See you in four months," but it comes out sounding hollow; false. We are all a little disturbed by the distance. I think it was difficult for those we left behind. I was going so far away, and may be gone before they could see me again. I don't like seeing this thought reflected in my family's faces as we load up the car and drive away. I will miss the dogs, who seem confused but comfortable staying at my parent's house. I hope they will be OK while we are away. *All* of them, canine and human.

We arrive in Columbia, not really knowing what to expect. We check into our hotel, and all any of us can do is sit and wait. We have meetings with the doctors and other staff starting early in the morning. We sit, we wait. Nobody sleeps well.

THE WELCOME

We make our way to the fifth floor of the Richland Memorial Cancer Center. As the elevator door opens, I am struck by one thought: we are in a special place. The large front desk is bustling with activity. Emblazoned in bold letters on the soffit over the desk are the welcoming words, "BONE MARROW TRANSPLANT." I am shocked—an entire *floor* dedicated to the one treatment I need. My confidence is immediately bolstered simply by reading that sign.

We meet one of the five doctors who run the medical aspects of the BMT unit, Dr. Godder. She is, I can tell, a powerful woman—not in terms of politics, but in her knowledge, control, and intelligence. I like her immediately. She has the rare ability to be two people at the same time: the caring optimist, and a no-bullshit clinician. She reviews my case with me, asking the usual medical questions relating to last bowel movement, whether I smoke, and my previous chemotherapy. She also, however, asks things like, "How long have you been married?" and "What are your dogs' names?" She laughs at my admittedly stupid jokes. Her eyes sparkle with enthusiasm; she clearly loves what she is doing. As I said, I like her immediately.

She gives us her analysis of my situation, and after detailing the vast multitudes of fatal complications associated with the transplant process, she tells me, straight up, that I have a 15, maybe 20 percent chance of survival. My biggest risk factor was (and still is) relapse after (or during) transplant. Typically, adults with relapsed, refractory B-cell lineage ALL have a 35 to 40% mortality rate due to complications during transplant.

Essentially, I had about a 60% chance of making it through the next month. I liked those odds (even if they didn't necessarily apply to me).

We have been thinking that Pit would be the donor, but it turns out that my mom may be a better candidate. She and my father shared one antigen type, and I had inherited it. Instead of a 3-of-6 match, as I had with Pit, we had a 4-of-6 match. Nobody knows if that is better, and the doctors all shrug, but we all like the sound of it. We quickly discover that experimental treatment involves more unanswerable questions than known entities. Answers to questions are frequently prefaced with phrases like, "We think..." and "It may..." and *always* end with "...but we don't know for sure. All we have now is a theory."

During this time, I am fitted with a "pick line" which is a tube that hangs out of my arm and is used for blood draws, chemo infusion, and transfusions. The line that is already in my chest apparently doesn't have enough ports. I get to watch, fascinated, as the surgeon feeds it into the vein. After pushing in about eighteen inches of tubing, the end is near my aorta, and he stitches the "outside" end down. The nurses later are thrilled that it has been stitched, as many unanchored pick lines ended up "falling out," the remaining infusion (whatever it may be) draining onto the floor.

We all agree that I need to undergo pre-transplant chemotherapy to lower my tumor load, which already is off the scale. If I do not, the sudden overload of dead cancer (and formerly healthy tissue cells) will likely block the vessels in my liver, killing me. Once my marrow becomes inactive (again) I will go into conditioning therapy (chemo, radiation) for the transplant, which I will do behind the airlock, in the BMT unit. This will likely add another two to three weeks to our stay in South Carolina. All we need is insurance approval. I pass all of my pre-treatment tests (without the benefit of insurance), and am pronounced fit to handle the rigors of transplant.

We meet many other patients, both pre- and post-transplant, during the various tests. John is on Day 33, and his 30-day bone marrow biopsy shows that all is well. His wife, Nancy, wishes us all the best during transplant.

John sounds good, and appears fairly healthy. Thirty days post-transplant seems so far away. Pat is 36, has AML, and wants to check out my pick-line, as he will be getting one placed later that day. He seems a little squeamish, so I spare him the details, telling him that I didn't really feel a thing. Deborah, wearing a mask, sits in a wheelchair, her 3-year-old daughter climbing all over her. Dan, her husband, stands watch over the scene. Pat, Deborah, and I probably will be entering the airlock within a few days of each other. All I need is a "yes" from the HMO.

Unfortunately, the insurance company is dragging their feet, betting that if they drag them long enough, I will die. Their bet, in too many cases, is a good one. They stand to save hundreds of thousands of dollars by delaying my treatment. I wonder how they sleep, if they sleep. I am beyond anger, nurturing a quiet, white-hot, glowing rage. I envision my future, chained to Health Net's corporate headquarters, with a sign that reads, "Health Net is killing me by denying me care." Those bastards will have to cut the chain after I am cold, blue, and stiff. Maybe then people will see human beings, not dollar signs. I am not an "inefficient use of resources," as one report from the HMO's "panel of experts" states. The person who made this statement, in their "thorough" review of my case, referred to me twice as "Doug" and once as a female, Mrs. Collins. Makes you wonder just what field these fuckwads are "experts" in.

In my educated estimation, without treatment I have about three weeks to live. The approval process often takes months. The concept of stress, as in "the stress of driving in traffic" takes on a somewhat different meaning. The walls are closing in around me, and all I have the power to do is wait...*wait.*

We wage our battle from a small, second-floor kitchenette perched above the highway. Carol handles most of the campaign (wisely keeping my foul-mouthed rage away from the phone), recruiting Congressmen, news anchors, and lawyers for our side. In this battle, she is as dangerous as a grizzly defending her cub. The HMO initially denies coverage, then delegates the heel-dragging to the "appeals" process (which, basically, is a legal route the HMOs take to delay care as much as possible, hopefully long enough for the patient to die waiting). Carol made it clear that I was going forward with this transplant with or without insurance coverage; that wasn't going to stop us. Then, Dr. Godder takes them on. I don't have any idea what she said to them, but soon after they rolled over and approved, even before they had finished the appeals process. I said it before, she is *powerful*. Carol, Dr. Godder, and Pat, the insurance specialist, make one hell of a scary team, if you are in the health insurance industry. I couldn't be happier to have them on *my* side.

We blaze over another hurdle, sprinting hard again as we hit the ground. I am to check-in the following morning to begin pre-conditioning chemotherapy. I cannot see where the hurdles end, but none have tripped me yet. I am the luckiest man alive.

Welcome to Chemo

I am somewhat stunned by the nurse's first topic of discussion. After introducing herself, she shows me the two "hats" that are placed in the toilet. One in front for pee, one in back for crap. All I can think is, "God, the indignity...the horror...the embarrassment...the *smell!*" I can't imagine choking down dinner with a full one of *those* adding ambiance to the room. I ask, almost pleadingly, if this is really necessary.

"Yes, it is. We need to measure everything that goes into you and comes out. By the way, unless it's an emergency, don't vomit in the toilet. We need to save that, too."

"Can't you just take my word for it?"

"No. When you are finished, just call the front desk and let them know."

Egad.

I am infused with a mix of chemo drugs; some are new, and some I've had before. One of the new ones, Ifosphamide, requires me to pee at least 150 milliliters every hour, on the hour, for two days. To accomplish this daunting task, I drink huge amounts of fluids, and receive a liter of saline every three hours through my IV. I manage to sleep 15 minutes at a time, then am awakened by a smiling nurse waving a urinal. After 48 on-the-hour pisses, I am allowed to sleep.

I respond as I often do to chemo—sleepy for a few days, but feeling pretty well. My magic formula for remaining well consists of three components: Eat as much and as often as I can, exercise, and drink at least three gallons of water a day. There is a stairstepper in the hallway, and I hop onto it at least once a day. I do laps with Carol around the unit. I do everything I know to remain well through this part of the treatment; if I falter now, it could kill me in the next couple of weeks. I must stay strong, healthy, and keep my attitude up.

News arrives from the hospital in San Francisco. The jubilant Transplant Coordinator explains that a perfect six-out-of-six match has just turned up on the global registry. The possible donor lives in Germany, so the marrow would need to be flown, with a medical escort, as soon as possible, to San Francisco. I am now blessed with another option! We are all excited, and initially pursue this new, miracle match with all of our collective energies. We soon realize that, although it is a miracle, it is an impossibility¼.

The problem is the time factor. Everything my body is telling me indicates I can't keep the fight going much longer. My estimate is that more chemotherapy to delay transplant, *might* keep me alive for another six weeks, *if* I am lucky enough to avoid opportunistic infection. I also feel that any additional chemo I undergo will help my already-resistant leukemia become more powerful, more difficult to eradicate. I cannot find a doctor that will argue with me. We (me, Carol, and the SC team) discuss all of the various consequences of each course of action with experts on both coasts, and are left in the middle; each group has its own institutional bias and wants me in their studies. I somehow must separate opinion from fact. The only way to do this is to ask.

The minimum time that the average global bone-marrow donation process takes is two months. I would need to fly back to San Francisco, *sans* immune system. I may die from an unseen disease or mere cold circulating throughout the fuselage before I even make it to the transplant center. But first, the entire process must be approved by the heavy-footed insurance company, who interpret our urgency as a reason to step slowly and ploddingly. Meanwhile, I would be given one, possibly two more high-dose therapies in order to give every entity involved the time they need. I would be waiting, unprotected—a ripe target for any common bacteria, virus, or fungus to attack, for an absolute minimum of three weeks; realistically more like *ten*. Over the last two years I have learned to take all the advice, weigh all the options, then go with my gut instincts. My gut is screaming, waving its arms and stomping its feet, insisting that I stay put, and follow the first course of action, already accepted and embraced.

I tell Dr. Abyankhar ("I-be-on-car") of my decision. He breathes an enormous sigh of relief; he had remained a neutral referee, not offering any opinions, only listening and nodding, offering unbiased facts, as I debated my fate. With a relieved smile on his face, he excitedly says, "You have made the right choice!"

I, too, am relieved. I am making my own decisions, which the people here not only encourage, but require. The staff give patients a palpable feeling of control. It is, after all, *my* disease, *my* treatment, and *my* life. The decisions, therefore, are mine. This is how medicine should be practiced *everywhere*. The ability to steer as the ride hurtles unpredictably along is important; it provides confidence, without which I'd already be ashes.

Dr. Abyankhar brings in a pile of consent forms, each related to a different experiment, clinical trial, or study. The results of these extra tests and procedures will be used to further the growing knowledge of treatments, and help them manage the side effects of BMT more effectively. Some require blood draws, some are tests with drugs, placebos, and different dosages, and some need an extra draw of bone marrow. Everything taken from me is to be studied, each with the possibility of filling potholes in the road I am now traveling, making the ride smoother for the passengers behind me. Carol and I read about, discussed and decided to participate in all trials I qualified for before we got there. So, without hesitation, I sign every one of them. Dr. Abyankhar, grinning, breaks into amazed laughter. He explains that most patients are unwilling to undergo additional testing and experimentation, and my eagerness to be involved is unusual.

I am floored.

How the hell do other patients think their own, possibly life-saving, treatments have been discovered? Improved? Focused? Do they realize that, a mere ten years ago, their disease was a death sentence? Do they realize how *little* they have to give, and how much can be gained? Given this chance to regain life, it is my fundamental *responsibility* to give back, to honor the sacrifices of the thousands before me, who so altruistically gave of themselves in an effort perhaps to save mine. It is a duty I cannot imagine trying to escape. I have been given so much. To ignore the souls of those who fell on the front lines or the needs of those who will come after me is unimaginable. They will learn from me.

As in previous high-dose regimens, my white blood cell count quickly drops off to almost zero. We aren't going to wait for it to climb, however. When it hits its lowest point, I am transferred into the mysterious area behind the airlock to begin my conditioning therapy. I am happy beyond words to be actually here, ready for transplant, facing *life*.

INTO THE AIRLOCK

Conditioning Therapy. So innocuous-sounding. Seemingly painless. I guess "Retching Therapy" wouldn't bring in so many volunteers.

Regardless of the name they give to the often-fatal doses of chemo and total body irradiation, I can't wait to get started. I have to convince doubtful nurses that I am happy to be getting a bone marrow transplant. We had to bite, scratch, and fight to be here, and are quite pleased to have made it to this stage. I guess many people aren't all that pleased to be in the bone marrow unit, or to be receiving this treatment. I can't relate. I, as with everyone else here, would be dead without it.

I arrive in good shape; the BMT unit is maybe thirty yards from my initial hospital room, but it is really a world away. A world that I will be locked in, maybe for just a short time in my life, maybe for the rest of my life.

Roger, Carol's father, mails us a laptop computer he found at a used electronics store (my hands are numb with nerve damage from the previous chemo, and I am unable to manipulate a pencil). I am grateful to be able to write down whatever enters my chemo-pickled brain. It's a great way to get everything that is spinning around in there *out*, thereby dramatically increasing my chances for sleep. I feel like there is already much I have forgotten, and need to catch up on documenting this experience.

I am to begin conditioning treatments in the morning. Carol and I settle in, ready to run headlong into the next battle.

The efficiency and skill of the team (which is really a *team*, not some illusive "concept" dreamed up by a seven-step weenie management guru) astounds me. Nurses, doctors, pharmacists, nutritionists, social workers,

55

and insurance specialists work as a coherent group. Each of them knows exactly what is going on with every patient's care at all times. Information flow is swift, and action in a crisis is immediate. I still cannot believe that a corporation had anything to do with this place. It runs too smoothly. They all are committed to one goal: life. This group of people simply does what they are trained to do, as well as they know how, and the bullshitting, profit-minded, time-wasting bureaucracy is where it belongs—out of the equation.

Yes, I'll be the first to admit it—thinking about the evil specter of corporate America and its large population of asshole MBA's leaves me feeling like I have a chalky, bitter pill stuck in my throat. They tried their damnedest to allow the cancer to kill me off before I could waste any more of their money. The BMT team put the patient first.

Nurses here only work on the bone marrow floor; rotations from other floors are nonexistent, so these people are specialists. The team of doctors passes information on patient status, and discusses treatment options on a regular basis. Ego, apparently, never interferes. Neither does the almighty dollar. Essentially, every decision made had six specialists backing it up— me, as well as the other five doctors. I never needed a second opinion, because I already had five. I never doubted any conclusions we reached together, and never second-guessed anything.

This is how medical care should be. Carol and I are *so* glad to be here.

GIFTS AND GRATITUDE

While we are busy mapping out my present and future medical care, some longtime family friends are putting together a fund-raising effort, to offset the steadily rising costs of our little endeavor. Spearheaded by Susan and Karen, it is sure to be a success. From the time I was a baby, just about every holiday from Thanksgiving to Easter has been celebrated with Karen, Susan, and their families. They *are* family. Just north of them, in Burlingame, high school and family friends of Carol's also launch a fund-raiser at Our Lady of Angels church. They are an enthusiastic 20s and 30s group rallying behind us; some of the guys even shaved their heads in solidarity!

Carol and I are blown away by the unsolicited show of support. We are also a little reluctant; we have never been the focus of so many people, many of whom we have never met. Our faith in the goodness of the human spirit is bolstered and set in stone as donations roll in. I measure the quickly-growing fund not in dollars, but in the growing feeling of caring, nurturing, and community that will carry us through our hazardous adventure.

The fund-raisers are more successful than anyone ever possibly imagined. The biggest part of the success lies in my own realization of how many lives I have touched, and how these multitudes are now coming together for one goal—to help save my life.

Carol's co-workers also amazed us with their generous donations of hard-earned vacation time. They gave us their time off so Carol can be with me. What a gift!

I find it difficult to express how deeply this has affected me and Carol. I am being carried out of a burning building by *hundreds* of compassionate rescuers, not left to fry in the flames. How can anyone fully express their thanks for so many selfless acts? I promise myself I will find a way to let the good that has been given to me grow, and be spread around. They will learn from me.

CONDITIONING

I am physically and mentally well going into Conditioning Therapy. My faith in the staff, and in my ability to withstand the rigors of the impending chemo and radiation, is running high. The risks associated with transplant are, to me, inconsequential. Remaining alive while killing the leukemia is the only goal that means anything to me. Cataracts, sterility, liver and kidney failure, diabetes, heart failure, infection, pain, rejection, graft-versus-host disease, secondary cancers, brain damage, lung damage, pneumonia, fatal hemorrhage and anaphylactic shock are non-entities. I never consider any of them as risks. They weren't important, because they weren't killing me now, and may never even happen. Leukemia is killing me *now*, and I need to kick it out of my system. Forever. *Now.*

In my visualizations, Meme is no longer surfing through my bones. I am there, alone. Nobody to rely on, nobody to blame. Kill these little bastards. *Now.* My mind creates *frighteningly* violent images. Savage ripping and shredding of flesh. Flying bits of brain, bone, and warm sprays of blood. Screams of pain and surprise. Limbs torn off and twitching, painting the floor with their fleshy, spurting ends. All this gore and violence by my hands, *with* my hands. The miniature, wrinkled personifications of the cells that are my disease are trapped. Nowhere to go. Pleas for mercy only make it worse. One by one, I hunt them down, armed with a clawhammer. I split their skulls, crunching through steaming red guts as the claw end strikes home. I thumb eyeballs until they burst, squirting thick, whitish rivulets of goo all over my forearms. I bend elbows backwards, standing on their shoulders, until they snap like chicken bones. I wade through the mutilated bodies as I eagerly, *droolingly* pick out my next screaming volunteer. I am perversely enjoying myself as these scenes play themselves out in my mind every night. They will *suffer* for what they have done to me and the people I love.

> *My ANGER*
> *SWELLS inside of me*
> *I'm taking it all out on you*
> *And all the SHIT you put me through...*
> *NO ONE here is getting out alive...*
> *This time I've really lost my mind and I don't care*
> *so close your eyes*
> *and kiss yourself goodbye*
> —Green Day, from song "*Having a Blast.*"
> (one of the aforementioned angry punk bands)

Every morning I am led downstairs, out of the airlock, to receive the total body irradiation. I stand against a wall, like a knife-thrower's target, and am dosed, from head to toe, with heavy radiation. My lungs are shielded with lead, to avoid scarring them to the point that they would no longer work. I am to remain completely still. If I move, the radiation may clip the edges of my lungs, frying them irreparably. As with my previous radiation, I can smell a strange odor; the odor of heat, like the smell that happens if you leave a stove burner on accidentally. It's both a feeling and a smell at the same time. I visualize the leukemia cells vaporizing, leaving only shadows where they once stood. They do not even have time to run, as they try to do before I claw-hammer liquid-filled holes in their mis-shapen little skulls.

The technicians and doctors applaud my attitude, as well as my ability to stand still. Without exception, they tell me that I am the friendliest, most cooperative patient they have ever had. I find this strange and incon-gruous. Other patients apparently have been grumpy toward the very peo-ple who are trying to save their lives. I understand the need to be angry at *something*, but it doesn't make *any* sense to angrily slap the hands that will, with luck, pull you from the fire. I continue to be astounded by the care givers' ability to *give*, too often with only an insult or angry word as their reward. They deserve better.

Once again I am infused with the "piss every hour for two days straight" type of chemo. Just as I near the end of the 48 hours, my lungs fill with fluid due to the merciless hydration through the IV line. I am, in effect, drowning. My blood pressure skyrockets. My oxygen saturation level, normally high, plummets. I am dosed with diuretics to make me piss out the excess fluid, am fitted with an oxygen mask, and gulp numerous blood pressure regulators. Both sides of my body are strapped down with IV lines, and I must keep my bed in an upright, seated position to keep from drowning. I can actually *feel* the fluid slosh around in my lungs as I readjust my position occasionally. Night and day have lost all meaning. I am not allowed to sleep; each time I start to nod off, my breathing slows, and my oxygen saturation level plunges downward. I must wake up and consciously force myself to breathe deeply to remain alive. It is the most exhausting exercise I have ever done. I have to concentrate all of my energy on constantly breathing as deeply and heavily as I am able, and I haven't slept in 48 hours.

I have a sudden, all-encompassing, *violent* need to get the *fuck* out of there, to leave, to *run*. I feel like Gulliver, every limb tied down, unable to move. Something in my brain, driven by an enormous, suffocating claus-trophobia, snaps. I reach for the mask, and yank it off my face. I can feel my eyes bugging, my pulse hammering, and the prickly, itchy sweat on my neck. My next impulse was to rip the IV lines out of my body, and get *out*. Carol and the nurse physically hold me down, waiting until I am back in control. The nurse, Una, calmly forces me down, hands on my shoulders. In her deliberate, Southern way, she says, "We're all goin' t' get through this, Dave, so you may's well just take it easy an' relax." When I quit strug-gling, quit trying to rip the lines out of my chest, she injects a double-whammy of Ativan. Gradually I calm down and regain command of the stifling, strapped-down-with-a-wet-itchy-blanket feeling. I stay in control, breathing deeply, sitting up in bed, and do not sleep for another two days. Finally, just hours before the actual transplant, the fluid drains from my lungs and I can rest. I am frightened by the fact that I had lost control. I was ready to rip the lines out of my veins, tear off the mask, and *run*.

When transplant day arrives, I am more exhausted than I have ever been. After 96 hours of chemotherapy, without sleep, I am unable to fully appreciate the incredible physical and spiritual process of regaining life, of feeling life refilling my body. I yearn to be *present*, to welcome the new life, but I can only lie there weakly, detached and inert. It is bitterly disappointing to feel so uninvolved, when I had *so* wanted to be an active participant. It is like getting picked last for the kickball team.

Welcome Home

Our mantra for transplant day is "welcome home." It is our way of greeting and accepting the new marrow. Mike (my nurse) brings the plastic infusion bag in, full of MA's treated marrow, and I am awestruck by its incredible, almost neon pinkish-purple color. Somehow, actually *seeing* life in that bag gives me a preternatural flush of energy. The marrow has an inner light, all its own, that is unique and special. I envision my marrow spaces as freshly cleared, richly dark soil, fertile and warm, where the marrow will grow readily and happily, producing flowers of the same, pinkish-purple light. I am tired, but I will live. They will learn from me.

I will live with this incredible light inside me, and will let some of that light out into the world where it can be seen and appreciated by everyone. I sleep, oblivious to anything but the beautiful, glowing flowers, which send their roots branching deeply into the rich, welcoming soil of their new home.

MY SLEEP GUARDIAN

Although I encouraged Carol to go to the apartment at night so she could rest, there were many days before and after transplant that she (fortunately) refused, and she became what I soon referred to as my "sleep guardian." She would snooze during the day, while I was (generally) awake and relatively functional; she would then show up in the evening to watch over me. I was entirely protected and at peace when she was on sentry; every time I stirred, she was there, smiling at me, ready to pull me through what may come.

Each time I woke up (every two hours or so), she would, in a blur, unplug the six IV pumps, get my slippers, and guide the whole ensemble of weak, dizzy, bald guy and interminably beeping machine to the bathroom. While I was busy blasting out yet another hot frothy jet of diarrhea, she would scurry out to alert the nurses that it was time to take care of needed charting, meds, or vitals. I would already be awake, and would once again be gracing them with a full "hat" for their inspection.

For the first time in five days, I actually slept for three hours straight! I slept as well as possible in the hospital, as she minimized all of the inevitable (as well as necessary) intrusions during my nights. Vital signs taken every two hours, various medicines administered in between, and the panicky, nonstop trips to the bathroom normally make it impossible to create space for sleep, but Carol organized and managed everything so that I was probably the best-rested patient on the floor. Just getting all of the IV lines untangled and machines unplugged took me two minutes if I was alone. Two minutes is an eternity to one with stools as thick as your average cup of coffee, and thankfully Carol was there to ease me through the nightly routine.

She rubbed my legs to send me back to sleep, and pulled me back to wakefulness when ugly dreams reliably appeared. She held the basin while I puked myself dry—heaving painfully, gasping for breath, and wishing there was something left to dilute the bitter bile. Productive puking is much less painful than the choking, gasping agony of repeated dry retching. Carol was right there with me, feeling my grief as if it were her own. She kept the IVs running, soothed me to sleep, and quietly and lovingly stayed by my side, urging me forward. Watching me sleep peacefully was the only reward she wanted; the only one she asked for.

I don't know what I ever did to deserve her, but it must have been something *good*.

LIFE BEHIND THE AIRLOCK

Two days after actual transplant, the maximum impact of ten days' worth of chemo and radiation finally hit me. The fastest-growing cells in my body (cancer, digestive tract lining, new skin, and hair) are killed. To my amazement, thick callouses on my feet and hands simply fall off, leaving thin, painfully sensitive pink skin behind. The skin on my tongue, as well as the lining of my mouth and esophagus peels off in whitish sheets, leaving the flesh beneath raw and exposed. The pain is solid, dense, suffocating, especially when taking oral medications. Swallowing feels like a truck is driving slowly over my chest. Sipping a little water results in a deep, powerful sting that cause waves of dizziness and occasionally makes me vomit. I maintain my mouth care routine, knowing that the pain of brushing skinless gums is preferable to a fatal infection. I do what I must to survive, as I always have. But soon I am unable to say more than a few words. My mouth and throat are a giant, open wound. I know that I am in the worst of it; things surely will get better.

My skin turns bright red and begins to flake off in hard, reptilian scales. It feels much like a blistered sunburn, one that keeps you awake at night with its hot, prickly itch. I am covered with dark purple bruises, due to the combination of low platelets and ceaseless subcutaneous injections. Everywhere I have received a shot erupts in a quarter-sized purple bump. My shoulders and thighs are almost solidly bruised; fortunately, the bruises do not hurt, they are just a little grisly-looking. Carol is immune to these now, unphased by what once paled her. Various steroids, at high doses, cause fluid to accumulate in my legs, ankles, cheeks, and torso. The thin, peeling skin is turgid and stretched, like an overfilled water balloon.

Holding anything down becomes a challenge. I want to continue eating, to keep the juices flowing, but my digestive tract is no longer able to process anything properly; it often rejects what I try to pass through. Every time I have to take the oral anti-fungal liquid (three times a day), I need the basin by my side, ready for action. The horrid flavor of this stuff would make a goat puke. I struggle against my stomach's protests, holding it down while trying to keep the pain at bay. I *must* hold it down, as it protects me from potentially lethal fungal attacks. I am motivated, and am usually successful.

My brothers fly out for a visit. I feel a strange responsibility to not let them see just how rough the road has gotten, but I realize they already know it is a difficult period in the transplant process. I know I am lucky; I am simply experiencing normal post-transplant recovery, and have no significant complications. The afternoon they arrive, I am in quite a bit of pain, mostly in my chest; the lining of my stomach and throat, ruined by the chemo and radiation, is sloughing off. Despite my efforts, I spend a miserable portion of their first day in South Carolina doubled up in bed, heaving. A large, slimy sheet of something finally comes up. It is part of the inside of my stomach, white and torn. It looks (and feels) like peeled-off chicken skin, and my brothers appear repulsed and fascinated at the same time. Their foreheads wrinkle with concern, but they pass the basin back and forth, studying the contents and making comments. My throat feels (and, actually, is) shredded, the lining hanging in ragged scraps like rotting curtains. Fortunately, an increased dose of morphine starts working its magic. Things get better; the truck stops driving slowly back and forth over my chest and neck, and I can now divert my (slightly dopey) attention to just hanging out. I am grateful that I can gather the energy to share a laugh or two with my brothers. They are clearly happy to see me, doing what I must, and doing it well.

Finally, due to immense, overbearing pain, I am unable to eat anything, and go on intravenous "food" (a.k.a. TPN). I also agree to a morphine drip, which makes it possible for me to *talk* again, relatively pain-free, for short periods of time. Occasionally, the morphine isn't enough to veil the pain, and I need to get a little "bump" to make the gauzy fabric between me and it just a little less translucent. Pain is a funny thing. You often don't realize just how much you are experiencing, and how it dominates your reality until it is suddenly diminished. The feeling of freedom is beyond words. Having pain go from omnipresence to mere annoyance is liberating. I feel like a *person* again. The hurt never *really* goes away, but sleeps fitfully as the painkillers are increased.

The IV "food" actually boosts my energy level, and I manage five or ten unsteady, heart-pounding minutes on the stairstepper most days. My brain tells me exactly what the body needs, even as it whimpers in protest. I doggedly crawl over to the machine, start the timer, and go. Sometimes I last ten minutes, sometimes thirty seconds, but I *go*. I must keep my abused body healthy during recovery. Nurses and doctors praise my efforts, calling me "compliant." I only comply to what I know will keep me alive. I am *educated,* not compliant—I know what will work for me, and use all the energy I can summon to do all I can. If I am to die, it won't be because I gave up. I will die in the act of *killing* my cancer, not being taken *by* it.

The morphine drip eventually manages my pain well enough to *try* eating; unfortunately, my interest in food returns much faster than my physical ability to actually process it. My failed attempts invariably become successful regurgitations. I stubbornly try eating every day; one cannot define one's own boundaries without bumping against them now and then. I know that I must collide with my limitations as frequently and vehemently as possible. Eventually, they will be pushed outward.

> *Do what you want*
> *do all you can*
> *break all the fucking rules…*
> *and die like a champion*
> *ya hey*
> —Bad Religion, from song *"Do What You Want."*

By this time, Carol has met quite a few other patient's families out in the hallways where I am not allowed. She learns that Pat, a patient I met earlier has been transferred to the ICU, with uncontrollable hemorrhaging. He is bleeding from every orifice, draining as fast as they can pump more blood back into him. Things did not look good; one of my doctors said that if people went to the ICU they often didn't come back. I send Pat and his family all the good energy and hope that I could, secretly and guiltily thankful that it wasn't *me* in there.

Another patient, a Mrs. Collins (a strange coincidence of names) was also in the ICU with unspecified complications. The expressions on the nurses' faces when I ask about intensive care, tell the story. It is the roach motel for bone marrow patients. Check in, but don't check out. Most of the unseen, anonymous patients just on the other side of the walls around me were still, like me, managing to stay well enough to avoid intensive care. If I had one fear, it was of being sent down there. It was a death sentence placed on the dying. I made it a goal to never to be on the same *floor* as the ICU.

MIKE

Mike was usually my daytime nurse. We were quite similar in our frequently infantile sense of humor. He was a five-year veteran of the BMT unit, and had his job well-handled. Many BMT nurses burn out quickly from the pressure, the hours, or the horrors they face every day (which no doubt haunt them long after bedtime). Mike seemed to thrive on the energy, good and bad. I never saw him make a mistake—except one. Somehow he got the idea that he could, maybe, *somehow*, repulse me. He gave it his best. *My* mistake was to think the same of him. I, too, gave it everything I had.

Mike, like me, thoroughly enjoyed a good, disgusting contest in which each participant would attempt to out-embarrass or out-gross the other. We would employ every weapon we could and both of us were frighteningly well-armed. Second-grade level bathroom humor; lots of references to the rectum and its output; long, detailed discussions about color, texture, and volume of body refuse. Neither of us ever won.

Mike, as a bone marrow transplant nurse, had seen and experienced a dazzling array of truly hideous bodily functions, secretions, and bedpan deposits. I, as a highly decorated hospital veteran, had not only created my own dazzling array from time to time, but also have experienced the in-your-face embarrassment of a plethora of uncomfortable situations. Rectal exams. Testicular exams by a female doctor with my mother in the room. Daily stool samples. Uncontrollable diarrhea farts with a room full of visitors. Crapping myself because I couldn't unravel the IV lines fast enough to get to the bathroom. Enemas. A nurse exclaiming, "Your anus is very pink, Mr. Collins," loud enough for friends waiting outside to hear.

Numerous bowel-related discussions with friends or family or both in the room. Spread-eagle naked testicular radiation in front of a large, open doorway to a common hallway. The technician, a woman trying in vain to preserve *some* dignity by speeding things along, asked in a heavy southern drawl, "Mr. Collins, will you please hang onto your penis? It keeps falling in the way." An as-yet-unidentified man came in, and exclaimed, "Well, isn't this nice? How are you, Mr. Collins?" I replied, "I'm just hangin' out!" He laughed, then made a speedy exit.)

One would think I had the overwhelming advantage in any "most embarrassing moment" or "gross-out" competition. Such was not the case.

Mike is the only person I have ever met who could not only keep up, but holds his own in the bathroom-gross-out genre. He had a story to match every disgusting and embarrassing anecdote I tried on him. He never even blushed when I told him that the radiation fried the skin on my nuts to the point that they looked as if they had been coated with Col. Sanders' secret recipe. Didn't flinch when I told him that the crispy coating fell off a couple of days later, a scrotum-shaped crust that floated in the toilet and proved to be a difficult flush. He smiled wryly as I described my new "invention," designed so that we BMT patients wouldn't have to get out of the recliner to take one of 20 or so foamy, liquid shits each day. He even enthusiastically made suggestions as I described the apparatus, which involved a five-gallon wet/dry vacuum, a snug-fitting silicone "seat" attached to the hose, and a buzzer that signaled discreetly when the unit was full.

We called most contests a draw.

I had previously warned you that my "embarrassment line" may be somewhat blurred; perhaps it's invisible. And if you are still reading at this point, you will realize that I was serious. Anybody want to have a "gross-out" contest? I'll smoke any challengers—except Mike.

Not only did Mike's disgustingly juvenile sense of humor mesh very well with my own, but it also was a *great* foil for the oppressively stressful, mind-numbingly frightening life behind the airlock. Few people I know can transition into laughing during potentially life-threatening circumstances, but he did it flawlessly. He would say things like, "Your platelets are down to 4 today. I'm getting a transfusion for you soon, but you can't hemorrhage between now and then, OK?" Once, he burst in, all excited, and exclaimed, "You're up to six liters of diarrhea today!!" "If we take you off the anti-diarrheal, maybe you can beat the all-time record of eleven liters! I'm up for it if you are!!" I wasn't, but I appreciated the thought. My *God*, eleven liters…almost three *gallons*. I'll bet that record will remain unbroken for many years to come. I wonder if they gave that guy some kind of trophy.

Occasionally, Mike needed reprimanding, so I'd threaten to crap myself, smear it all over the walls, and he would have to clean it up. He'd threaten to "open up a big ol' can o' whoop-ass" on me. Among our master-plans was to get a fresh, unused "hat" (those toilet devices), put some snack-pack chocolate pudding in it, and talk Carol into snapping some pictures of us spooning up and devouring the "feces." Future plans for these pictures included the hospital's bulletin board. Maybe even the hospital newsletter. Perhaps I'd mail a few to the HMO to show them what they were spending their half-million on. Alas, those plans never reached fruition. Mike and I certainly had a lot of fun, even if everyone else in the room was gagging.

LIFE RETURNS

It is day +10 and my new bone marrow shows faraway, faint signs of life! My white cell count, which has been zero (indicating no marrow activity), goes up to 0.1 (normal range is around 8.0). We are excited, but at the same time full of dread. One *very* important question remains: is the activity shown by my blood counts generated by M.A.'s marrow, or by remnants of my leukemic marrow that somehow followed me out of conditioning? When I close my eyes, all I can see inside me are the wonderful, neon flowers produced by the new marrow—not a scraggly weed in sight. We can only wait, buoyed and supported by the wishes and prayers of the people in our lives. I believe, with each strengthening beat of my heart, that the leukemia is gone.

My white blood cell count, with the help of growth-factor injections, slowly climbs. If it steadily creeps above 1.0 for three days, I will be allowed out into the hallways. For now, I am content to pump away on the stairstepper, which has found a permanent home in my room (I am apparently the only person on the floor with any interest in using it), and sit upright in the recliner. Pneumonia kills many post-BMT patients, and I am determined to keep it at bay by expanding my lungs every day. I also believe that a fast-beating heart gets the blood going too fast for the shit that could attack me to gain a foothold—bad stuff flushes out faster with increased flows through the filters. My little theories may not be medically accurate, but they serve me well.

I would enjoy reading, but my short-term memory is shorting out. I forget what I have read, even as I am reading, and I get confused very quickly. I turn back pages, reread paragraphs, and skim previous chapters, trying to reorient myself. I cannot even keep characters straight. It is maddening. I seem to remember things that never happened, and forget things that happened two hours ago. Carol shows me pictures, taken a couple of days earlier, and nothing rings a bell. I have no recollection of posing for them. I forget conversations with friends and family in California, and am frustrated when people recount things that I previously talked about. Too frequently I cannot recall a goddamn thing. The staff tell me that this is common, and *usually* gets better with time. It scares the hell out of me to imagine that they could be wrong, that this could be permanent. I imagine that this may be something like having Alzheimer's, surrounded by the fear that the world could be cruising away without you. Maybe forgetting things is the natural defensive action of the overloaded mind—like a heavily burdened truck, stuff just seems to dribble right off the top as it travels along; the bumpier the ride, the more falls out.

The nurses are efficient, friendly, and extremely capable. They deal with *real* emergencies every day, calmly, skillfully, and professionally. However, one nervous nurse-in-training makes one of my mornings white-knuckle frightening. It is her first day trying to fly on her own, without any supervision, and she obviously has been pushed out of the nest with more down than feather. She is jittery and unsure of herself. I can *feel* her getting more and more flustered as she makes error after error, and I realize I am beginning to panic right along with her. Too late to do anything about some of her errors, I sit and fester. I am to be doped-up on Benadryl soon. How the fuck am I going to keep an eye on her then? I hoped, Susan (the charge nurse) would be hawking her for the rest of the day. I had no choice but to defend myself against her, as the mistakes she made with my care could potentially kill me.

I am too upset, too shaken—walking the sharp edge of panic. I placed my life in these people's hands, and up until this morning, have unquestioning confidence in their skill. I need to regain the feeling of trust; this whole thing will fail without it. Carol arrives just as I finish a tirade and she takes control for me. Trainee-nurse comes in to infuse my Benadryl, and pushes the needle into my central line without cleaning it first. We both stop her from continuing; any bacteria on my port would be pumped directly into my bloodstream if she were allowed to proceed. I am now angry, but I am also *scared*. Her lack of attention and skill could kill me!! Carol orders her to pull the needle, leaves the room, and quickly returns with the charge nurse. She has pointed out the mistakes that need correcting, and demanded the trainee no longer be allowed in my room. The trainee appears shattered. I feel a little sorry for her. She is in this business because she *cares* about people. I, however, must be able to trust my care givers; to trust them with my *life*. Given these stakes, her feelings *cannot* be considered. The bone marrow unit is no place to make a mistake, and she has gone well over her limit with me.

Mike and Kathy, most often my daytime nurses, are now to be my *only* daytime nurses. I am relieved beyond words, as they are skilled, knowledgeable, and unshakable. They *are* people with whom I can trust my life. Carol and I are grateful that people with their capabilities exist, and that they have dedicated their lives, existing for *me*.

Inching Forward

I feel a little improvement every day, and begin to take in small amounts of food. My body's stubborn rejection of oral nutrition begins to wane; soon, I am able to eat an occasional bowl of oatmeal, or an instant cup of soup. I am motivated by my need to feel aware, to try to wean myself from the morphine, perhaps a little too quickly. At times I need an extra shot to keep me from screaming in pain and frustration. I do not enjoy the foggy, half-consciousness that morphine sometimes brings; I want to be sentient every second that I am alive. I understand how a person *could* get hooked, as the sometimes searing emotional pain is erased just as quickly as the physical. It creates a sheltered, protected bunker, burying the pain under heavy, deep layers of earth. An inviting way out, I'm sure, for many. I, however, want to experience everything that I can, in whatever time that I have. I am acutely aware of the ephemeral nature of consciousness, and desperately want to preserve each moment. I want to *clearly* see what is down there while I stand on the edge. I also can feel that my liver and kidneys are tiring. They have been putting in some serious overtime cleaning out the toxins, and deserve a long, chemical-free vacation.

I stay on the IV food, as I am not yet eating meaningful quantities. I have lost quite a bit of weight, and want to hold onto every ounce I have. The fewer I lose, the less work it will be to regain my strength. My confidence grows as the worst of the side effects begin to wind down. The doctors seem pleased with my progress. One simple fact continues to motivate me, and keeps my eyes intently focused on the road. They are, at this moment, *learning* from me.

76

On Day 18, my white count bravely peeks above the magical level of 1.0. The new marrow has engrafted! I leap over another hurdle, sending up sprays of gravel as I land, already racing toward the next. At this rate, I may be released from the unit by Day 28! We are encouraged and optimistic as my body, nurturing new life within, repairs itself. My food intake increases rapidly, and I am able to hold down at least two small meals each day. I continue to climb onto the stairstepper every day, and I am actually feeling human, within my own body, most of the time. Earlier, I often felt unattached to my physical body. I could feel what it was going through, but it felt secondhand, like I was experiencing the various side effects with somebody else's body. I have no lingering fevers, I am finally off of the morphine, and tomorrow I plan to stop the TPN. My IV pole, once laden with six pumps, is stripped down to two as I am weaned from around-the-clock drugs and hydration. It is much easier pushing it across the floor to the bathroom, since it now weighs about a third of what it once did. I am happy to have been given the chance to get this far. If I had listened to the doctor in San Francisco, I would have died five weeks ago.

Dr. Godder is pleased as well. On Day 20, she not only frees me to walk the halls, but in her blunt, no-bullshit manner, informs me, "You will be released tomorrow. I can see no good reason to keep you here. Tomorrow at ten A.M. we will have your discharge conference." My mouth gapes in disbelief. I was mentally planning for discharge (at the earliest) ten days from now. Carol has ten days' worth of preparations to make in the next 24 hours. She attacks her assignment with a happy fervor, working through the night to prepare our new home.

I walk the narrow hallways, mask and IV as my companions, feeling an amazing freedom and sense of *space*, despite the fact that the hallway is only about 50 feet long. As I am entering the kitchen, Pat's wife and sister come out of his room; they look worn and haggard. Pat is obstinately hanging in there, tenuously clinging to life. Elizabeth, his wife, says with a smile that he squeezed her hand today—a sign that he is on his way back. He has been unconscious in the ICU almost as long as I have been in the

BMT unit. They have stopped his near-fatal, uncontrolled bleeding, and plan to send him back to the unit soon. They were there to make sure his room was ready to receive him. I am happy for them, and for myself as well. People can tell you the odds, and you can beat them. Pat's success proves the probabilities do not apply to everyone, maybe only the people who believe in them. After all, I had been called a "statistical zero," and I was still here. I chose to believe that statistics did not necessarily apply to me. *I* am different.

Seasons merge seamlessly. Through the narrow window of my hospital room in Sacramento I had watched the shimmering heat of summer become the crisp, bracing cold of midwinter. The new year has come and gone, and I find myself here, *alive,* in South Carolina. Winter, progressing silently outside the large window of the bone marrow unit (observed but never felt), has passed like a shadow. I am being released as the first Spring blooms tentatively peek out of their seemingly dead branches. Life is returning, full hope and color, from its cold, gray slumber.

THE APARTMENT

Before I got the pre-transplant dose, Carol had managed (with the help of Pit and the BMT unit social worker) to rent an apartment that has been specially cleaned and furnished for bone marrow transplant patients. I had stayed there one night before chemotherapy began. Now it looks strangely cavernous. I have gotten used to living, eating, sleeping, puking, and exercising all in one twelve-foot-square room; by contrast a 1000-square foot apartment is almost too large to comprehend—for about three hours. Then, the walls start to close in. I want to be out and about very badly at this point, but have been sternly warned not to go anywhere, or do anything except make the thrice weekly, ten minute pilgrimage to the BMT unit for bloodletting and subsequent testing. Our new schedule is difficult to follow; I have trouble (due to chemo-brain) even counting my pills out correctly. Suddenly being in charge of everything is gargantuan; frightening, as any screw up or oversight could dislodge large, overhanging boulders, sending their grinding force rolling straight for me.

The new environment, still very isolated, has its own, daunting list of do's and don'ts. The first weeks on our own, left to administer meds, IV fluids and electrolytes, blood growth factors, and injections, are dizzying. Each individual step we take must be precisely timed, precisely administered. Any deviation from our strict schedule could have dire consequences. My difficulty lies primarily in short-term memory lapses, induced by the chemotherapy. I count pills, lose my place, and have to start over many times. I forget that I have already done certain treatments, and get halfway through filling syringes before I realize that I did this already, a few short hours ago. We eventually write everything down, step-by-step, so that neither one of us lets something slip by. Carol may not have had the brain-freeze induced by the chemo, but functioning at peak levels is impossible. We are both frustrated by our inability to fully comprehend and remember things, despite the reasons why.

LIFE ON THE OUTSIDE

My risk of fatal infection is high; I am nervous, suspicious of everything. Within a few short hours, an unnoticed or untreated infection could easily take over my body, infiltrating major organs, causing them to sputter and fail. I could be dead tomorrow from something secretly incubating inside me, taking advantage of the lack of barriers to its growth.

It is a time to be careful.

We have taped the fireplace shut with plastic and mailing tape—it is a major air leak to the forbidding outside world. I cannot cook—a burn easily could become infected, or I could bleed severely from a simple cut. I cannot handle anything that is uncooked—bacteria, particularly e-coli thrive on fresh produce and meats. I cannot even touch plants outdoors since any fungus or bacteria on the leaves could send me back into the hospital. I wash my hands, scrubbing away invisible killers, if I have touched anything, even a doorknob. I imagine my hands swarming with infection from opening the car door, washing them as soon as I walk in the door of the apartment or the BMT unit. I cannot read the newspaper—virulent fungi and parasites lurk in the pulp that the paper is made from. I read mail wearing rubber gloves, having been warned that viruses can stay alive for *days*. I wonder how many people with dripping, infectious colds handled this envelope before it reached me? How many phlegm-filled coughs has it absorbed? How many people blew their noses, then grabbed this package and sent it on its way? My old world no longer exists. It has been swallowed by an enormous, deadly creature that may still be lurking about. I must be watchful to avoid being greedily devoured.

Very few people can comprehend this intense need for absolute cleanliness and isolation. Some react by rolling their eyes, assuming we are just being paranoid. "Oh, you don't *really* need to avoid children, do you? What if you already had kids?" Others condescendingly look for apparent inconsistencies, and point them out to us. "I thought you couldn't get near raw vegetables…how come you can eat a carrot?" We patiently explain how diseases are commonly spread, why my immune system is not presently functioning, how susceptible to everything I *really* am, but it is frustrating as hell. Some people take us at our word, but each rule must be justified over and over to those who won't.

I don't like to think this way, but I get the feeling some people call so that I can make everything right for *them*, to put my hand on their shoulders and reassuringly murmur, "Everything is fine. I am totally normal again, and we can all resume our lives as we have always lived them. It's all over now." But usually, when I'm insistently grilled, I want to scream, "I don't fucking know if I'm going to be alive at *dinnertime*. Quit asking me to tell you that I know more than that, because I don't." The phone rings, and I involuntarily become defensive, regardless of who is calling, or why. I realize that they want to help, to send me all the good that they can, but I am *tired*. I cannot continually defend myself against death, and justify my behavior regarding what is necessary to keep me alive. If all my precautions involved medicine instead of behavior, people wouldn't even question it. "I take a pill so that I don't get chicken pox from an unknowingly contagious child," is more tangible to most than the reality which is, "I must avoid children for at least two years. I have no defenses against the diseases that they often, unknowingly, carry. Your little pox-covered angel, without even a touch, can kill me."

Suddenly, everybody seems to believe that behavior isn't important. This is the core of the frustration that I feel. My *behavior* has been the reason I have stayed alive until now. I am following the rules that I know will keep me well, keep me *alive*. I resent the cross-examinations and doubtful, unbelieving responses to my new life requirements. *Yes*, for the fifty-thousandth fucking time, it really *is* this strict. I eagerly accept and live with the damage and bitter losses I have sustained. Why can't you?

LOSSES

I am not one to focus on the losses that cancer can bring, but losses do need to be acknowledged. People on the outside, who haven't been exposed to this type of experience before, focus on the tangible losses: Hair. Weight. Jobs. In their effort to comfort, to help, they manage to focus on those sacrifices which, to this cancer patient, are low on the list of what really matters, what makes our lives enjoyable and productive.

Cancer ends friendships, stealing the unconscious ease that people once had to be themselves in your company. It raises sharply barbed barriers around you, imprisoning you inside, alone, with its jagged, bloody edges. Cancer erodes physical abilities and independence, and forces one to ask for help. It steals one's ability to earn their keep, decreasing self-worth. It takes away dignity and privacy, leaving feelings of invasion and nakedness. It erases memories, burning them away from the conscious mind, leaving only smears and shadows in the space they once occupied. It creates upheaval and anarchy in a formerly predictable life, creating confusion and despair. It singles you out, causes you to be somehow different; then people treat you as an outsider. You do not any longer belong in the normal stream of life. It causes sterility, ending the dream of raising a child who has your eyes.

Focusing on surface losses, like hair, understandably is about as far as many people can go. However, this narrow vision ignores the deepest insults: in order to survive, intangible parts of your life must be dropped unceremoniously into the abyss. Too often taken for granted, many of these lost facets of richness and meaning will *never* come back. Much of our recovery goes on inside our heads; the physical aspect is easy. Not much energy is needed to grow hair. Carving a new world, one in which we are comfortable, fulfilled, accepted, and equal, is the challenge. We not only have to discover where we want to make those first, tentative moves toward shaping a new space for ourselves, but must invent the tools with which to form and mold the spheres of our lives. Some of us make it. Many don't. I am on my way.

GAINS

Cancer is not powerful enough to take everything. Many facets of self remain, and many more emerge, previously hidden, or maybe newly carved. These are priceless artifacts, buried in sand and gradually exposed by the raging winds, just waiting to be gathered, cherished, and appreciated. The strength of family is bolstered and solidified. Faith in the goodness of humanity, and the depth of the heart, are renewed and reinforced as acts of kindness and compassion pour in from unexpected places.

Many people, once involved with your life, *do* fade into the background, but for each relationship lost, there are many that appear, coming out of shadows and into the light. It is the truest test, and the people who remain by your side when the dust begins to settle are those you *know* you can trust with your love. Doors close, but more open. As we gain strength and confidence, turning the knobs becomes easy and natural. As we reach for another to open, which may reveal new wonders, we find it easier to shut the doors to rooms we can no longer access.

We gain focus, the ability to assess what is *really* worth getting upset about, and are blessed with a unique and special ability to take each individual moment in life and appreciate it fully. To immerse ourselves completely, nakedly, in the pool of experience, and to never, ever again, doubt the inherent good that is at the center of every human heart. To *exist* in the present, while maintaining the ability to look to the future. To be a genuinely good person, a positive conduit for the flow of energy throughout the universe. To be given the strength to live without regrets, without the feeling that you should be doing something more, something different. To make *today* a good day to die. To gain fulfillment not with length of time, but with quality.

THE OUTSIDE, CONTINUED

Every other day, I strap on the mask (bright blue, so people are *sure* to stare), and Carol drives us over to the BMT outpatient clinic. I sign in, wait in the lounge (unfortunately, the only show the lounge TV ever has on is that fucking Jerry Springer, and its cast of lost, idiot souls), and eventually am called to the back to have blood drawn. Each step of the way, I am quizzed about bowel activity, urinary function, quantities, colors, and consistencies. Such questions, by this time, are part of normal life; they are all answered without hesitation, embarrassment, or regard to who else may overhear.

From the blood-draw, I am escorted to another room, to wait for results. Magnesium, potassium, liver enzymes, blood counts, cyclosporine, and steroid levels are all checked and adjusted as needed. Some days, I need platelet transfusions; some days, it's whole blood. Most days, I need potassium and magnesium, which I administer myself, in the apartment. The entire team—doctor, nurse practitioner, nutritionist, pharmacist, social worker, and miscellaneous med students—make the rounds, ensuring that nothing is left out, nothing forgotten. I am checked, head to toe, and pronounced fit to live for another day, with the stern admonition to call if there are any, even the most insignificant, developments in the next 24 hours. I strap the mask on, yet again, and we make the five-minute journey back to the apartment.

The feeling of freedom in that five-minute ride is lavish. So much *space.*

Arriving back at the apartment, I call the home-care company to let them know that I will be available to take delivery on the supplies I need for that day: syringes, floppy plastic bags of IV fluids, and injections arrive within the hour. Carol always answers the door. After the extreme isolation of the BMT unit, it is impossible for me to feel comfortable with people entering the apartment. Even a knock on the door is a frightening invasion; I must be on my guard all the time.

The IV pole is my constant companion; I am attached to it six hours a day. Its crappy little casters refuse to roll on the flat carpet in the apartment, so I am relegated to carrying the metal-and-plastic albatross if I want to go from the couch to the kitchen. It may be to my advantage, however; lifting that thing and holding its forty pounds while walking may be the best bone marrow patient exercise yet. Maybe, when Spandex doesn't sag on my bones, I'll make one of those obnoxious exercise videos. How to do crunches in a hospital bed, attached to six different IV lines, with uncontrollable diarrhea. I'll call it *"Sphincters of Steel."*

I spend countless hours looking out the window at life outside my new airlock. People going about their business, unaware that they are the object of my voyeurism. People are so unconscious of the *freedom* they have. They come and go as they please, walking their dogs, grocery shopping, getting the mail, heading toward the pool. Soon, each of the nearby dwellers has their own nickname: Frizzhead; Army Guy; Beagle Guy; State Trooper; Ponytail Flipper; Red-Truck Guy. The only regulars I know by name are Dan and Deborah (Deborah got out of the unit about the same time I did), who probably stare out of the windows of their own airlock, wondering when they can become a part of the stream of everything again. For now, time can only be spent watching life around us. Normal life is a spectator sport.

A lizard takes up residence on our porch (where I am not allowed), and delights me daily with his acrobatics on the railing, and his swift munching of anything crawling around that is smaller than him. He soon becomes Lenny the Lizard, and even Carol rushes over to check it out when Lenny makes his appearances. Sunbathing one day, Lenny apparently has his danger-radar off, and is messily devoured by one of the local cats. Briefly escaping, he runs across our porch, toward me. He had been bitten badly, smearing blood behind him on the concrete. As the cat bears down on him, Lenny turns, mouth open, and charges to attack, getting in one final snap of the jaws before the cat, tired of playing with him, chews him up and swallows his twitching body. If I go out, I'm going out like Lenny. Fighting every step of the way.

Two weeks after release, the doctors tell me that it will be OK to go to the mall, and get some exercise indoors before the stores open. I have never been aware of this interesting phenomenon; the mall opens early, just so people can walk. We decide to try it out soon after given the green light. It is a strange world of darkened storefronts and competitive seniors, throwing their elbows up high, breathing in through the nose and out through the mouth, and deliberately picking up speed to pass you if you are in their way. Scornful looks are thrown at those who do not yield to the speed of the power-walkers. Unwritten mall-walking laws must stipulate that slower traffic keeps to the right, against the closed stores, because the speed walking, cane-toting seniors glare at us if forced to pass on the right. It's like driving in impatient traffic.

Despite its downside, mall-walking does have its benefits. It allows me to exercise, gives me a little space, and is relatively safe, as there are few people actually in the malls at seven A.M. I can easily tell when I am making progress, because I am able to do an extra lap, or go down the stairs twice instead of once. The woman who is always there walking, the one with the military swagger, the squeaky shoes, and the attitude, no longer passes me as if I'm standing still. She's lucky if I let her by once in two laps, and *she's* cutting the corners. We always leave as the mall's music system kicks into gear—the sign the stores will open soon, bringing the crowds I must avoid. Also, I have a firm belief that Kenny G. and Michael Bolton are bad for the immune system, and may induce vomiting.

Eventually I am allowed to walk, with mask, outside! It must be after the sun sets because sun exposure can cause graft versus host disease. Dan and Deborah join us occasionally, and soon our evening strolls become a three-or-four night per-week exercise. We begin to go for a few tentative dinners (we have, coincidentally, picked the same few restaurants as "safe": pizza, spaghetti, nothing uncooked or overly-fondled before presentation. It is refreshing to spend time with them; we are all around the same age and have many of the same griefs in our lives, not just the cancer. Just two couples, working hard to make a better tomorrow. We rent movies, play Uno, and generally have a good time, being people who may have *too many* inside jokes to share.

Soon, Dana's family (an 11-year-old with ALL) joins in the fun, as do Pat and Elizabeth. It is, after three months of near-total isolation, like finding a family ready to include you, and fully accepting of all the rules you need to live by. The problem with our new families, however, is that they often get sick.

They often die.

I began to worry about Deborah first, then Louise back home. Deborah lived just across the parking lot, so her arrivals and departures were predictable. When she left for a week, no word, we became worried. ICU? GVHD? HEAD INJURY? REJECTION? There is little to do but wait for rumor, or to see a family member. As luck would have it, Dan rounded the corner in clinic one morning, Maria under one arm, newspaper and coffee in the other. Deborah was ok. She had slipped, sustained an ugly hemorrhage on the back of her head, and some resultant clotting and vision problems. She would need to stay in the hospital for observations, since they were continuing to pump her brain full of anti-coagulants (to keep her safer from stroke.) Dan said she'd be likely to join us again in the next coming weeks. She peeked out of her room, looking somewhat cross-eyed and shaky. We waved back, trying to send her some hope, some happiness from the outside world. From where I sat, she stumbled and convulsed like Mohammad Ali, who once floated like a butterfly and stung like a bee.

Pat didn't give us time to worry; he pulled an endo over his walker, and got himself a shamelessly purple beet-shaped knobby-looking thing on his noggin, too. He, however managed his feat of strength in the bathtub. He really got those ambulances wound up as they blazed through the parking lot, sirens screaming wailing and everything. It was clear that Pat and Deborah's falls had scared Carol, so she made sure I had something to sit on in the shower. I was even humbled enough not to protest. My balance, admittedly, sucked, and I was numb from the knees down from some of the chemotherapy.

Louise's lapses between calls began to grow worrisome, however. I know that one of her ways to deal with gut-suckingly bad news was to clam up and do the deprivation-chamber thing. I did it, too. The last time I had heard from her, however, was two weeks ago. The longest she ever left me hanging was four days. I had 2,500 miles between us, no other phone, and all numbers were listed. One thing I never want to do is have a good friend bail out and die without letting them know that I love them first. I must get back to California, if only to brush back her hair, squeeze her hand, and tell her one simple phrase… "*YOU* mattered to *ME*."

Finally, Louise's daughter, Sherri calls. Louise is in China, attempting new, East-meets-West treatments for her abdominal cancer. Her western surgeon has given his OK to the Chinese to do a kind of 50-50 treatment, using all kinds of Chinese oils, herbs, foods, acupuncture and other un-Western advances to help her out. Sherri is the official town crier, to let us all know that all is well. We are, apparently, going to all ends of the world to continue our lives. Louise will be back, coincidentally, toward June, when I am likely to be back to Sacramento. It was exciting to think that we may, through all the battles in such faraway places, once again see each other, victorious and alive.

With our hopeful-soon release nearing, Carol and I begin to fit a few small plans for the return into the daily regimen.

MOVING ON

Just as we bone marrow patients feel well and confident enough to tag along with some of the world, to make some efforts at regaining life, we are told that it will soon be time to go home. It is exciting, to feel that we will soon be in our comfortable homes, enjoying our friends and families, doing whatever the hell we want, but it is also sad.

We have created our own, small society here amongst ourselves, with our own set of rules and taboos. Being thrust out again into the real world, to which none of us really feels attached anymore (we may even feel a little hostile toward it), subdues and fills us with more "what ifs." The sad truth, as Deborah said, is that the minute we feel good enough to discover each other as friends, we are taken away again by what remains of our old lives. We all continue to walk, to talk, and to squeeze what we can out of each day. We grow close quickly; the bonds forged from our shared experience are made of an amazingly malleable, yet impossibly strong ore, not often found and rarely put to the hammer.

Deborah, although she has a nasty graft versus host disease (GVHD) infection, makes the trip home first. Her doctor actually worked at the Richmond BMT and therefore could be trusted with her upgraded care needs. Dan calls a few hours after they arrive home; he tells Carol that a family of foxes moved into their backyard. They are happy to be there; we are happy for them. At home for one night, she is rushed to her new hospital. Details are sketchy. After two long weeks, Dan calls. She's alive, with severe GVHD and thrombocytopenia (a disorder of the platelets). We are unnerved, but happy to hear that she is still in the fight. Dan, also caring

93

for his two young ones, sounds exhausted. I admire the strength he must have to keep on. I guess that when called to do, some of us just do.

ALL FALLING AROUND ME

Deborah's death is quite a shock…not because she died, but because she went *home* and she died. It is very difficult to separate the two. So many others I had not met died soon after leaving. Pat had just been given the green light to go back, and now, unmercifully, traces of his old marrow show up on his latest biopsies. Taken from the anti-GVHD drugs immediately, he instantly gets the diarrhea, rashes, liver and kidney failure associated with GVHD. He is pissing blood, and from the chemo he may have developed enormous gallstones. His hair had just started to grow back, and he's back into the ICU. His liver is failing, and things do not look good. SHIT! We all worked so hard!

The latest news from Sacramento is not helping…Louise is having rapid, unexpected tumor growth, and is now in my old room, #214, at Mercy. I have been given the green light to go home, too. We make plans to leave mid-June. I can barely fathom a date that seems so far away, and can only wish for the best—that Louise will be there, alive and well, when I make it. There is nothing left to do.

THE LONG WAY HOME

We begin to make our preparations. It is amazing the amount we have accumulated in the last months. We decide to ship everything lightweight through UPS, and carry all the heavy stuff ourselves. Extras (cheap unfinished bar stools, kitchenware, towels, and bath supplies) we donate to the next BMT dweller. Even at $1400 a month, we needed to buy a few extras simply in order to make eggs in the morning! We hope the extras will come in handy for the next needy crew. We still have weeks before our return, but the preparation is immense. Before I can move back in, the house interior must be painted, scrubbed, ceiling scraped, HVAC system cleaned, vents sealed, HEPA filters installed, and all furniture steamed, recovered, or replaced. The carpets must be either double-steamed or replaced, and any curtains washed. I will arrive without any real immune system, and will be shuttled through the airport as quickly as I can be. The thought of so many people that close to me scares the shit out of me.

THE JOURNAL

8-10-98

Louise finally succumbed to the tumors that were ravaging her body (but not her mind) for so many years. I will always reserve a space in my mind for her, to keep my thinking on the right course, to keep my spirits up, and, as she did every day of her life, revel in the simple, real pleasure of being alive.

9-3-98

We got a call from Elizabeth, Pat's wife, two weeks ago. Pat died. I'm tired. The ride is often unpleasant.

9-27-98

I can't sleep (again). Tired of drugs, I always sleep ok after tapping away for a few hours, until my eyes are scratchy and swollen. I was lying in bed, remembering the intense sense of triumph and joy when the pre-relapse treatment ended. I felt like I could kick anything's ass; after all, I had just stared Death (the pussy) in the eye and that little piece of shit backed off and slunk away. I couldn't wait to get life restarted. Now, post-transplant, I am not as confident with getting life in general started again. I fear that the second I start to regain a semblance of normalcy (working, being allowed to handle feces, etc.), that black-hooded motherfucker is going to be there, and I'm going to have to drop everything and kick him in the nuts again. The last nut-kicking appears to have that scrawny asshole doubled up pretty good for now, but I really am tired of stalling forward progress, having to turn around and deliver an eye-popping groin shot just as I begin to pick up a little speed.

I basically am living from week to week; every CBC that comes back within my new normal buys me seven more days, and then I sweat out the next one. I really shouldn't worry so much, but I can't help it.

The dreams come at me night after night, seemingly endless, and encompassing a general theme. I'm being chased; pursued. One night, it's animals; the next, people. Always, however, my pursuers put me on the defensive, and I have to fight. I fight with every molecule, every spark of my being. I awake before I find out who wins. Still, the dreams come. Another recurrent theme of late has been the "sick person who insists on getting as close to me as possible." It's basically, I am sure, a reflection of the frustration I feel at being so different, with such different requirements than everyone else. I do not belong. I guess that this may also be a separate scion of the pursuit dreams—there's someone (or something) that I can't seem to get the fuck away from, that does not understand or care about my situation. My question is: do dreams result from what has been, is, or what will be? Are dreams a creation of reality? Is reality simply a reflection of our dreams? I better stop this. I'm starting to sound a little stony, and it's pretty fucking late.

Another thing I'm pondering is why I only feel like writing when it's very late. Privacy? Quiet? Right now, I don't know.

As you may be able to tell, I've been somewhat slightly depressed sometimes. Sometimes I wish I could sleep for the next five years, wake up, and KNOW that it isn't back, nor will it be back. I would know that I'm cured, and could go about the business of life. Having kids. Working. Eating raw vegetables. Enjoying every minute of every day, not spending so many of my precious minutes wondering; *wondering*.

Friends ask if we can go to weddings, parties, meet for dinner, etc. My first thought is, "If I'm still alive." I have never actually come out and said this; it has simply come to me as naturally as a parent would think, "If we can get a sitter," or a workaholic would think, "if I'm not out of town on business." Death has entwined itself in my entire thought process; it has become part of my life. Most people *think* that death is a part of their lives as well. It's not. Death becomes part of your life when it comes down to just the two of you, staring unflinchingly at one another, and you get the chance to tell him that you either welcome him, or that you would like him to go fuck himself. Death's presence in my life has given me the ability to appreciate moments that otherwise would have passed like shadows, unnoticed.

9-30-98

Blood in my sperm Sunday night scared the complete shit out of us. Thought it may be a harbinger of relapse. ohfuckohshitohgoddammitohmyfuckinggodamigoingtobeabletolivethroughanothertransplantfuck. That pretty much sums up my first thoughts. Monday morning, asked Dr. Q. He shrugged, said it happens all the time, and took a piss sample. We left for the cabin later that day. WHEW!

10-4-98

Met Tish and the entire Norton clan. Wonderful to be alive to thank them all for the gift they gave Carol and me through the "Save Dave" fund-raiser. Good day.

10-13-98

More brain farts:

Top Ten Questions NOT to Ask a Cancer Patient:

1. "When are you planning to have kids?"—Out of the realm of my present reality.
2. "When do you go back to work?"—See #1, above
3. "Did you lose your hair?" followed by "Ohhh. That's horrible."—The losses that cancer brings are much more significant than hair. Focusing on hair may be convenient, but it insults the real losses. One loses longtime friends, jobs, physical abilities, body parts, and life. Permanently. Hair leaves, but it comes back. Yes, the pubes go too.

4. "When do you get out of the hospital?"—Only a time traveler can answer

5. "Are you cured?"—Even the most egotistical doctor can't call this one.

6. "When are you cured?"—See #5, above

7. "So you're all done, right?"—Cancer patients will never be "done" with cancer. It will forever be a part of their lives.

8. "How's the diarrhea?"—Do you really want to know? It's frothy, brown, painful, and constant. Sometimes, there's blood in it. Glad you asked?

9. "The whole family has the flu. Is it still ok to visit?"—Yes, if you are going to visit somebody else.

10. "How's your bottom?"—I'll speak for myself…the word "bottom" is childish. I prefer "butthole."

Victims and Victors

Don't *ever* insult me by referring to me as a "victim" of anything. I don't believe that there is such a thing if people are given a modicum of control over their life experiences as, or after, they occur.

I was watching the news recently, which featured a popular local teacher, proclaimed a "Cancer Victim" during the lead-in to his story. He had horrendous medical bills, two months to live, and his small community rallying around him. His two young sons sat anxiously beside him as the news crew descended.

NEWS: "How often, knowing what you're facing, have you looked in the mirror and said to yourself, WHY ME?"

CANCER 'VICTIM': "I have never, and will never, do that. I have so much good in my life. I have a wonderful family, great friends, a job that I love, and support from all over. I have never questioned any of the amazing amount of good that has come into my life; what would it be that suddenly gives me the right to question anything bad? I don't feel that I have that right."

I was stunned. For quite a while now, people have been asking me the same question, but I was never able to so eloquently answer them. This teacher, with his situation, gave US a gift. He showed us that despite what he faced, he would not do it as a victim. He has never met me, but he gave me a gift, too. He gave me a wonderful answer to this oft-asked question.

His seemingly ugly situation turned into something to be examined and admired. One may say that he is showing remarkable courage in the face of death; I disagree. He is showing us what is at his core—responsibility. Courage is not something to be "mustered," but is simply there, as a natural part of those whose inner core is built on personal responsibility.

11-8-98

Tomorrow I will have blood drawn to send to South Carolina for my 9-month checkup. I am not nervous about any problems, but I am somewhat out of sorts. It's just because, as Carol said, there is another hurdle to jump. It may not be as large as the many others I have cleared, but it is a hurdle nonetheless.

Dan called today. He is doing well (he must be if he is taking the risk of calling me, not knowing if I am still alive). He is managing somehow to keep his head above water, taking care of his two young daughters, working again, and living without Deborah to complete him. God, I admire him. I hope that he can take solace in the fact that one of our little family has made it this far.

11-9-98

No blood drawn today. Apparently, MedClinic doesn't stock the necessary vials; however, the hospital across the street, Sutter, did. The HMO, in their infinite wisdom, would not pay to have the vials shipped across the street, as they are not contracted with Sutter. Instead, they are going to pay for the vials to be shipped from South Carolina, to be filled with my blood here, in California, then shipped *back* to South Carolina, all of which will be done via overnight mail. Jesus fucking Christ. They cut staff to save money, then spend it on idiocy like this. It's amazing sometimes just how retarded the whole process has become. Give *me* the fucking money, I'll walk across the street, get the goddamn vials, and bring them back, free of charge. Just do *something* that makes sense. Well, I guess I'd never make it as a CEO. I still have some of my common sense intact.

11-16-98

Mailed, with Barbara's help, 60cc of blood to South Carolina for evaluation and testing. This past week has been spent a little nervously. Caught a cold, went on more antibiotics, but managed to come out without any secondary infections. Gab and Pit, meanwhile, were blessed with the arrival of Cleetus, (Justin Jon) on the 13th. We were planning to be there for the birth of the baby, but I'm no hypocrite; if I'm sick, I'm going to stay home. We now think we'll go on down for Thanksgiving, after all. I think the decision to go to San Jose is easier, now that people have something newer, and more exciting to talk about besides my latest CBC— Justin. Going then will also give Rog a chance to get over his (real, this time) cold. Fired the Rite Aid pharmacy today. They had a week to straighten out my prescription mess, and only managed to make it messier. The main problem was that if they couldn't, for any reason, fill the prescription, they just wouldn't, and would not even call me to let me know. Carol would then wait in line, and be told that it couldn't be filled because of (any lame excuse here). Today, I called them, and gave them the courtesy of telling the pharmacist why he was being fired. He went into a long list of excuses, whining like Dan Quayle, and never grasped the real problem: when my life-prolonging prescription is held up for any reason, I'd appreciate a phone call, so I can remedy the situation. I finally gave up because he just kept whining and that was getting old. My new pharmacy has a three-screw-up limit. Let's hope they manage to stay employed.

11-26-98

Thanksgiving Day.

Mowed lawns, cooked, spent T-day with Carol and the doggies. Many thanks, grateful to be breathing, aware, and ALIVE.

11-30-98

Back from long T-day weekend. Went to San Jose to see Justin, be with family. Went fishing for steelhead with Pit on the San Lorenzo River. Got a few small smolt, a few small rainbows on the roe that I had cured before. Drove back Saturday night, to beat the traffic.

Clinic today. White count up to 4.8 today. Neither of us was prepared for it to be that high yet. I spent the day trying not to think about it, waiting for the manual differential to come in, but thinking about it all day nonetheless. When will it be OK? When will I not worry about things? It's been three or four weeks of having unexplainable bodily reactions that I feared were relapse. Blood in sperm (leukemia likes to hide in the nuts), painful nipple, hard lump in chest behind nipple (lymphoma?) and now, today, an unusually high white count. I don't know if the stomach-dropping nervousness will ever leave. Maybe it's a good thing, a mechanism that is there on purpose—to keep me honest, to keep me thinking in the present. It's just hard to continually get the slap, "Maybe this is my last Christmas," kind of thoughts that come to me before I can block them from my conscious mind. They always hit on the blind side, when I'm looking the other way. I guess it's just something I will live with, like so many other things.

12-7-98

I don't know what to say. My white count is 10.4 today. It has more than doubled in the last week. I am very afraid that the cancer has returned. I made a call to South Carolina, to see if they have any of my 9-month shit back yet, but they will need time to get my chart.

I called Carol at work from the parking garage, unsure of what I was going to tell her. The good news is that all my other counts have also shown dramatic increases today. Hematocrit, hemoglobin, platelets all at record highs. Dr. Q told me not to panic until we get more test results back. We did a draw for a flow cytometry, but the results of that won't be back until later this week. My infection may have caused the elevated counts, along with the antibiotics, but I still am numb. I drove home from MedClinic with blurry, tear-filled eyes. I don't know how much more I can do. I don't want to leave Carol. I love her too much.

When I got home, I collapsed in the garage, hugging the doggies, who have no clue what is upsetting me. They look at me quizzically as I sit, face in my hands, wondering how I'm going to make it through this next trial. Even if the test results come back OK, these weekly scares are brutal, numbing, and oppressive. I want to hide, to remove myself from all that is around me, to crawl into a dark corner and hibernate until the harsh freeze is over. I think that I am close to the limit.

12-8-98

Slept (amazingly) well last night. I was exhausted. Our neighbor couldn't figure out what was wrong with her car, so I went over and fixed it. I needed the distraction, as I was hiding, trying to find the darkest corner I could, and doing something for someone else helped take me to a different place. I am doing OK today, more balanced, and can see that it is possible that I am not relapsing. All my other counts climbed, the infection started around 11-30, Thanksgiving weekend. I got antibiotics on 12-2, had a serious allergic reaction, and switched to another antibiotic on Tuesday. All of these factors can raise the white count. My differential is still normal, with a large increase in the percentage of neutrophils (a typical reaction to infection). Dr. Q, last night, looked at the blood samples himself, and saw nothing out of the ordinary.

Still, the overriding feeling is that I need to be doing something, to be prepared. All I can do right now is sit, wait, and try not to think, "what if…" Results will be trickling in over the latter part of this week, probably Friday. Waiting for the verdict is difficult, if I may employ a little understatement. I want to know now. The urgency to gather the forces for another battle only gets worse when there is really nothing that can be done. You can't get insurance approval for a procedure that may or may not happen. I'm tired.

12-9-98

Still waiting. Wondering. Speculating. Kevin called last night, didn't have the energy to pretend nothing was wrong. Told him the scoop, told him not to tell Rog. (Rog can handle the road, but only if he doesn't see the individual potholes.) Kevin seemed OK with everything, mostly shocked at the scares which have become so much a part of Carol's and my life, and that we generally keep hidden from everyone else. It's easier to learn about a scare after the fact than during so I keep information from leaking out and causing panic, and avoiding the phone calls in which I am asked to make it all better for the caller. Because I can't, I keep my mouth shut until final verdict. No sense freaking everyone out for no reason.

Called South Carolina myself and talked to Dr. Christiansen; all my tests from 20 days ago are normal. 100% donor cells. Can a person go from 100% donor to relapse in just 20 days? Why is my LDH high? Should I drop the Cyclo now, just in case? Is it significant that all my other counts climbed drastically, as well as the white count? How many more of these can I live through, before sanity pulls loose from its moorings? Maybe insanity would be easier. At least I wouldn't know what the fuck was going on. I would just live until I died, with no scares in between.

12-9-98 (evening)

Dr. Q called…not good news. I have some leukemic cells floating about. I knew what the verdict would be. I can already feel the pain in my kidneys and liver as the leukemia makes its way through my system. I stopped my Cyclo, and will be getting a biopsy early tomorrow morning. The plan is to let the GVHD take over, to see if it will kill off the invaders without killing me. I will follow this as far as I can take it. The next step after that will be the DLI. It will happen sooner if I have high levels of leukemia in my bone marrow. To answer the question, relapse can happen in two weeks. I have just proven this fact.

M.A. is driving up to give some blood samples, for testing. We plan to ship them to Sutter and to South Carolina, since we have no idea where we are going now. From the pain in my back and thighs, I can tell that there is something at work in there. Probably get the donor leukocyte injection sooner than later.

First call, Rog answered. He knew something was up. I just told him. Let the chips fall where they may. He was either in another world, or he was a rock. He took the information, asked what he could do, and generally was all business. No meltdown, no sobs, just wanting to know the plan, and what part he could play in it. People are amazing. You never know what they are capable of until you give them a test. Rog passed with honors.

Carol told me that whatever I choose, she will be there, right beside me, supporting any decision I make. I am in awe of her strength, her character, and her ability to stay in the fight. I love her more every minute. My only wish is, however this all comes out, there is love, happiness, and support in her life. She deserves it more than many. I am the luckiest man alive, to be able to spend my life with her.

12-10-98

Bone marrow biopsy this morning. Barbara came in, said she couldn't talk because it may make her cry to do so. Dr. Q also is upset. He has been in touch with the team in South Carolina, and they stress the importance of getting me out there ASAP. Due to the rapid, explosive nature of the leukemia, we all know that the marrow is going to be packed with it, even at this early date.

What we thought could be done here, in Sacramento, apparently cannot. I admit that I am disappointed; I don't want to go all the way out there again. It's so isolating. Leaving home again is difficult. If this doesn't work, we'll be out there, alone, in our own prison. I never want to go out like that, but I will if it gives me the best chance to eventually survive all this shit.

As I type this, Carol is getting plane tickets for next week, probably Wednesday. We will once again drop off the mongrels at San Jose and travel to the other side of the continent, since they are the only ones who can help me.

Anyway, I took the usual dose of morphine before, but it really didn't work this time. The pain was as bright and blinding as ever. I could feel my head and shoulders quivering as the needle sucked out the marrow. He had to take about 8-10cc, more than usual, so that may explain the excess pain. It's over, and the site isn't too sore.

12-11-98

It's official. I'm depressed. Last night I had a fever that I mistook for anemia. Was ready to cancel plans and just give up. It was a rush just to realize that a couple of Tylenol were all the treatment that I needed. I woke this morning, only wanting to go back to bed. I ate breakfast, sat around, and finally crawled back for a nap. Bad dreams. I beat someone who was bullying me so badly that his eye was hanging out of its' socket, his face torn from repeated kicks, and he could only lie in the street, spraying blood as he talked, telling everyone that I was the bully. Nobody believed my side, and accused me of being the asshole, and then I woke up. Has set the mood for the rest of the day, unfortunately.

12-26-98

I have chosen to quit treatment, and die at peace surrounded by those I love, and who love me. Most appear to support me in this decision.

Can you imagine, for a second doing anything, just cause you want to?
Well, that's just what I'll do so hooray for me
And fuck you.
—Bad Religion, from song *"Stranger than Fiction"*

If the leukemia was moving slowly, we could beat it with anything, but it came back so fast and aggressively I knew better. Another transplant quickly became my only option, and my gut didn't tell me that was what would work this time. My gut told me to stay home with Carol and the doggies.

Another day passes. Strange dreams as I doze during some of my drug-induced weariness. Today, I was taking colored sewing pins out of the backs of my hands, and punching them into the walls of the bedroom near the sliding door. No pain, just rearranging patterns and placing new pins. No idea what the hell it all means.

Rog, Roger, and Pit joined forces today to remove the horrid eyesore we called the deck. Looked like fun was had by all, and the yard looks huge! Hope I can stay with it long enough to make it look nice.

12-26-98

Strange new phenom…may be drug side effects. Words on screen do not exist as words on screen, 2-d, but as their own, individual entities. It makes corrections and reading difficult, but certain words appear to have more *in* them. It's impossible to explain.

12-30-98

This will be my last journal entry. I am centered, at peace, and I know that those around me will go on, and eventually will thrive again. I told Carol, in finding this peace, that I am not leaving. Where she finds a laugh, a smile, and happiness, that is where I'll be, and when she is ready for me again, and ready for happiness again, I am here in everything that makes her happy. I am happiness, and I am here. Always remember that. I love you. Thank you.

Dave

EPILOGUE

PARTING WORDS, THOUGHTS

I fear that over the last couple of years, I have witnessed too many eulogies read. Too many loved ones consoling each other, nodding in unison and agreement at what is said, and solemnly murmuring "It's true...that is what he or she would have wanted."

The speeches end; Glassy-eyed, like a worn-out herd of cattle, attendees make their way toward the sweating cheese and curling cold cuts.

As people solemnly eat, not noticing or tasting what has been supplied, they continually murmur about what the deceased would have wanted, nodding in agreement and picking their way through the darkening edges of the olive loaf and brittle baguettes gracing their plates.

It is during this time that I wonder...Who the hell *really* knows what old uncle Fred would have wanted?

To end the conjecture, I am going to tell you what I want, ending this age-old confusion.

WHAT I WANT FOR YOU

Realize the beauty of the moment, and *know* how lucky each of us is.

I want you to be your best, and to be honest with yourselves in your healing.

I want no guilt from anyone. You have been *important* in my life, so it doesn't matter what you called me in the second grade.

How each of you react to my death is *your* responsibility. Do not seek solace in a vice; I will *never* be available for you there. Please find the strength to make your response something beautiful and wondrous, and we'll all win.

I want you to raise your children to be responsible, caring adults. The world has enough victims. I want YOU to be a responsible adult, for the same reason your children need to be.

I want you to do something good for someone else, someone you may not even know, just for the hell of it, with no apparent reward for yourself. It may be the most important thing you have ever done.

I want you to remember me as you knew me, and don't glamorize me in my death. I was who I was, and death shouldn't change that. If you found me a good, honest, loyal person, remember me as such. If you thought of me as an idiot, remember me that way, too. Death does not alter what has been done in life.

Look for me where you find a laugh, a smile, or a good feeling. That is where I'll be, waiting to share it with you.

I have loved all of you, and I hope that my presence in your lives has been positive. Goodbye, if only for the moment.

-Dave Collins

AFTERWORD

Dear reader,

As Dave states in his preface, he was asked by many to write this book.. He in turn asked me, his wife Carol, to publish it for him knowing ultimately he could not.

When Dave was hospitalized I started writing and distributing an update letter that Dave and I continued together once he returned home. Those letters much to our surprise were widely requested and distributed by our family and friends becoming a source of strength, hope, inspiration, and humor. For this reason, Dave decided to write this book; in the hope that it could help people in some way.

Getting the book from myriad files and formats to publication has been a journey. Dave and I had support from many loved ones. My Dad suggested the book's framework which moved Dave directly to the computer to get started. My sister Karen, a former publisher/editor, finessed the work into manuscript format. Dave's brothers, my sisters, our parents, and great friends helped motivate me through my grief to publish his book. Mary Alice, Brian, Chie and Eric, Heather, and Evita among others kept me on the path with their enthusiasm and gentle inquiries. And in this final step of submitting the book to iUniverse.com, Marty has been incredibly supportive and encouraging. I am blessed with a life full of beautiful, caring souls.

Thank you all.

enjoy the day,

Carol Hewitt (Collins) Brej

More of Dave's photography and related links on the_ride.com.
http://homepage.mac.com/the_ride

ABOUT THE AUTHOR

Dave Collins, a vibrant young man, enjoyed life with his wife Carol and two dogs. He was a talented landscape designer spending most weekends fishing, hiking, or snow boarding from their cabin when diagnosed with leukemia. Empowered by his fighting spirit, depth of character, and colorful humor, he continued to live fully, love deeply, and inspires still.

0-595-21342-1

www.ingramcontent.com/pod-product-compliance
Lightning Source LLC
Chambersburg PA
CBHW020257290526
45784CB00003B/1280